PHYSICAL ACTIVITY AND HEALTH:
AN EPIDEMIOLOGIC STUDY
OF AN ENTIRE COMMUNITY

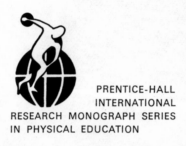

PRENTICE-HALL
INTERNATIONAL
RESEARCH MONOGRAPH SERIES
IN PHYSICAL EDUCATION

H. Harrison Clarke, Chairman of the Editorial Board

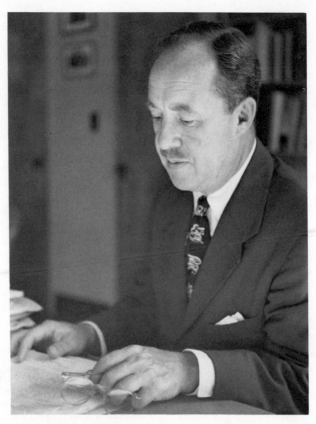

THOMAS FRANCIS, JR., M.D., 1900–1969

Dr. Thomas Francis, Jr., was, until his death, director of the Tecumseh, Michigan, Community Health Study. Early in his career, a talent and interest in scientific investigation brought Dr. Francis to the Rockefeller Institute, where he concentrated his efforts on infectious diseases, virology, microbiology, and epidemiology. In 1947 he was appointed to one of the first distinguished professorships at the University of Michigan, the Henry Sewall University Professor of Epidemiology. Although Dr. Francis maintained an interest in clinical medicine, research was his forte. One of the highlights in the career of this outstanding scientist occurred when he was entrusted to design and conduct the evaluation of the Salk polio vaccine. This exemplary double-blind field study, probably the largest medical experiment in history, attested to his genius as an investigator.

A few years later Dr. Francis turned his talents and imagination to the study of chronic, noninfectious diseases. His dream of a community serving as a research laboratory in which to study the impact of genetic and environmental forces on health and disease came to fruition in the Tecumseh Community Health Study. Fortunately, Dr. Francis recognized the importance of including habitual physical activity and work capacity among the factors to be studied.

Dr. Francis's depth of understanding of health and disease, his insight into experimental design, and his ability to quickly ferret out important details were clearly evident to those of us who worked with him on the Tecumseh Study. His friendship and guidance have enriched immeasurably my own personal and professional life.

H.J.M.

Physical Activity and Health: An Epidemiologic Study of an Entire Community

HENRY J. MONTOYE

Professor of Physical Education
The University of Tennessee

Prentice-Hall, Inc.

Englewood Cliffs, New Jersey

Library of Congress Cataloging in Publication Data

MONTOYE, HENRY JOSEPH.
    Physical activity and health.

    (International research monograph series in physical
education)
    Bibliography: p.
    1. Exercises—Physiological effect. 2. Physical
fitness. 3. Tecumseh, Mich.—Statistics, Medical.
I. Title. [DNLM: 1. Health. 2. Physical education
and training. 2. Physical fitness. QT225 M798p
1975]
RA781.M62   613.7   74-2479
ISBN 0-13-665604-8

Printed in the United States of America

10   9   8   7   6   5   4   3   2   1

PRENTICE-HALL INTERNATIONAL, INC., *London*
PRENTICE-HALL OF AUSTRALIA, PTY. LTD., *Sydney*
PRENTICE-HALL OF CANADA, LTD., *Toronto*
PRENTICE-HALL OF INDIA PRIVATE LIMITED, *New Delhi*
PRENTICE-HALL OF JAPAN, INC., *Tokyo*

*Dedicated to
my wife, Betty*

Contents

Preface

A muscle that is exercised becomes stronger. A person who undertakes a conditioning program increases his work capacity. More than a century of scientific study has left no doubt that an exercise program improves one's ability to do exercise. But does it do more? Will changing from a sedentary to a physically more active life affect one's health?

The notion that regular physical exercise may delay the onset or progress of disease is not new. However, two developments in recent times have made this controversial question more significant. First, modern technology has altered most of our occupations and modes of transportation so that we are now required to expend much less energy in our everyday activities. Therefore, if a sedentary life contributes to ill health, the evidence should be more manifest now than ever before. Second, chronic degenerative diseases have replaced infectious and contagious diseases as principal causes of death. It is logical to hypothesize that physical inactivity is more closely associated with chronic diseases than the diseases formerly responsible for most deaths.

One approach in the study of physical activity and health is the classical experimental design; namely, introducing an exercise program in one group of subjects and not in a control group. This is still the method chosen in some instances. However, in studies with human beings, unlike animal investigations, it is often impossible or prohibitively expensive to impose an exercise regimen and maintain the research design for a sufficiently long period of time to observe the effect on health.

Another less costly approach is a longitudinal observational study of a population living in a natural community. This monograph, for the most part, is comprised of data collected in a study of this kind. A relatively large number of people is involved; hence it would be classified as an epidemiological study. The word epidemiology, like epidemic, is derived from two Greek words, "epi" and "demos," meaning "upon or among the people." The Tecumseh, Michigan, Community Health Study, of which the present investigation is a part, exemplifies the literal meaning of the word, because the data were collected in, and represent, an entire community. Observational studies such as this are also not free of difficulties. The development of disease (or maintenance of health) is the result of a complicated interplay of many genetic and environmental factors. Hence, it is not easy to ferret out the cause-effect relationships, even with modern sophisticated statistical techniques. An epidemiologic study can be expected to generate some hypotheses about physical activity and health, rather than provide definitive proof of relationships. Hence, if this monograph presents some challenges, raises some questions, or suggests some important problems to be studied by other methods, it will have served a useful purpose.

For the most part the data which form the basis of this monograph were collected and analyzed under Grant Number HE-14712 (formerly CD-00246 and HE-12755) from the National Institutes of Health, United States Public Service (H. Montoye, principal investigator). However, the work was also supported by the Tecumseh Community Health Study Program Project Grant, HE-09814, from the National Institutes of Health (T. Francis, and later F. H. Epstein, principal investigator).

Most of the data contained in the monograph have been published in greater detail in various technical journals. The publishers of these journals have kindly granted permission to reproduce some of the graphs and tables. I am also indebted to the many co-authors who collaborated in the published papers. These include: Walter D. Block, Benjamin N. Chiang, David A. Cunningham, Stephen Dinka, Jr., Horace J. Dodge, Frederick H. Epstein, John A. Faulkner, Mary E. Frantz, A. Roberto Frisancho, Gordon E. Howard, Millicent W. Higgins, Sharon Guber, Benjamin C. Johnson, Andrew J. Kozar, Jacob B. Keller, Helen L. Metzner, William M. Mikkelsen, John A. Napier, Lawrence V. Perlman, Guy G. Reiff, Richard D. Remington, Ronald J. Saunders, Hugh G. Welch, Park W. Willis III, and James H. Wood. The frequent "skull sessions" we had in preparing the papers expanded my understanding of health, disease, and physical activity. Although the late Dr. Thomas Francis, Jr., Dr. Norman Hayner, Dr. Leon Ostrander, and Dr. Betty Ullman are not included as co-authors on any of the papers, their judgment and insight, nevertheless, were invaluable. I am also grateful to Miss Carolyn Carpenter and Miss Elaine Dempsey, R.N., who did most of the day-by-day treadmill testing; Joseph Consani, Nelson Meade, and Mrs. Martha Theros for their administrative help;

Gary Wilke, James McIntyre, Mrs. Alice Exelby, Mrs. Catherine Meade, Mrs. Ann Pfister, R.N., and John Mullin for their efforts in the field laboratory; and Mrs. Sharon Franklin, Mrs. Barbara Godfrey, Miss Candace Notestine, Miss Helen Smithson, and Mrs. Linda Weinberger who typed most of the manuscripts and reports.

HENRY J. MONTOYE

PHYSICAL ACTIVITY AND HEALTH:
AN EPIDEMIOLOGIC STUDY
OF AN ENTIRE COMMUNITY

Chapter 1 / The Tecumseh, Michigan, Community Health Study

The late Dr. Thomas Francis, Jr., renowned Professor of Epidemiology at the University of Michigan, viewed disease and disorder as the result of inadequate adjustment to factors in the environment (129). As early as 1940, he envisioned a study of an entire community—not just the people living there, but the biological, physical, and social environment and how these factors interact to enable some individuals to maintain health and others to be susceptive to disease.

The Study of an Entire Community

An ecologic investigation of an entire community, as contrasted with a sample of a population, has the following advantages, in the opinion of Dr. Francis (128):

1. The embracement of entire neighborhoods in juxtaposition to one another so that clustering of cases would be more readily discernible.
2. The continuous observation of comparable kindreds under similar environmental exposure is more readily maintained.
3. The detection and measurement of environmental changes and their effect upon health and pathological reactions can be more easily studied, since they can be more readily applied in a community than to items of a sample.
4. A continuous surveillance of the community of this size at least is more adequately maintainable than a geographic sample of a large population.
5. The effect of "community reactions" on health and disease

1

incidence are more likely to be measurable with respect to factors such as unemployment, elections, exposure to new highways, and epidemics.

6. Since a large body of data will be available regarding the community, a variety of relations can be examined or suspected ones can be tested without requiring separate or numerous ad hoc inquiries of each. Moreover, their validity can be readily checked in the same population or known segments thereof. One may thence develop hypotheses in the course of the study. Speaking of economy, one may ask how many ad hoc studies are equivalent in cost to one integrated study, or in their value to etiological analysis.

7. The entire complex of interrelationships between events, exposures, habits, and disorders can be explored. Similarly, the occurrence of different disorders in the same kindreds or groups may give information of common factors in etiology or response. This does not seem to be so readily approachable in a sample.

8. Since the studies require close integration of epidemiologic and clinical procedures with fundamental laboratory research, the location should permit ready movement of research activities back and forth, from the field to the clinic, to the laboratory, or vice versa, so as to develop methods of investigation and to permit their test under field conditions. Community medical facilities can be more effectively employed in the study of a total population than under sampling conditions.

9. I believe the examination of a population can under these circumstances be done less expensively than the study of a similar sample in a large city.

Tecumseh, Michigan

In 1957, with financial support from the state of Michigan and later from the National Institutes of Health, the dream of Dr. Francis became a reality. At this time, Dr. Robert J. M. Horton undertook the task of finding a suitable community in which to launch such a study. Tecumseh, Michigan,[1] located 55 miles southwest of Detroit and 27 miles southwest of Ann Arbor, was finally selected.

Why was Tecumseh selected for the investigation? Its size was an important consideration. There were about 9,500 inhabitants in this study area (approximately 56 square miles) with approximately one-third of the residents living outside the city limits. This population was large enough to produce significant findings and yet small enough for the project to be manageable. The community was sufficiently close to Ann Arbor and the University of Michigan Medical Center that travel would not be difficult, yet sufficiently distant so as not to be unduly influenced by the university environment.

---

[1]The town is named for the famous American Indian Chief and hero of the War of 1812. Chief Tecumseh was killed by troops under General (later President) William Henry Harrison along the Thames River about 150 miles northeast of Tecumseh, Michigan, near Chatham, Ontario.

Tecumseh is located in a rural, agricultural setting; hence, farmers and their families comprise a significant portion of the study population. Nevertheless, there are large and small industries in the area encompassing diverse occupations and a variety of socioeconomic groups. Good health facilities were available in the town and the population was not highly transient. Finally, and most importantly, the community leaders, members of the medical profession, and other residents of the community were civic-minded and favorably inclined to support the study.

A brief description and history of the community as presented by Napier, Johnson, and Epstein (270)[2] follows:

> Tecumseh was formerly quite rural in character but, like many midwestern communities, has been undergoing a fairly rapid industrialization. Its largest industry, Tecumseh Products, is the largest manufacturer of refrigeration compressors in the world. In 1966 General Motors opened an upholstery plant within the study area, and the Anderson Division of the Stauffer Chemical Company opened a plastics plant adjacent to it. About 40 percent of the labor force hold white-collar jobs, such as clerical, sales, managerial, and professional positions. Of the 60 percent in blue-collar activities, over two-thirds hold skilled or semi-skilled jobs in manufacturing. Approximately one-third of these industrial workers are employed by Tecumseh Products, while the remaining two-thirds are distributed over a wide variety of other enterprises. In all, Tecumseh has about 150 private businesses dealing in a wide range of goods and services.
>
> According to the U.S. Bureau of the Census, the city of Tecumseh had a population of 4,020 in 1950 and 7,045 in 1960. The size of the entire study community was not known until the completion of a private census in the fall of 1957. At that time the study community had a population of 8,787, of whom 6,246 were residents of Tecumseh City and 2,541 were living in the rural fringe. By 1967 the population had grown to approximately 9,800, made up almost entirely of Caucasians, mostly of northern and central European extraction. There is only one Negro family and there are about 30 families of Spanish or Mexican descent.
>
> From 1830 to 1930 the population of Tecumseh Village grew very slowly—from 1,727 to 2,456 persons. Since the establishment of its major industry in 1934, the rate of population increase has doubled during each census period: 19 percent from 1930 to 1940, 38 percent from 1940 to 1950, and 76 percent from 1950 to 1960. Since 1930 Tecumseh's population has nearly tripled in size, a growth rate considerably higher than the national average. In recent years there has been an influx of workers from larger urban centers seeking employment opportunities.
>
> Compared with places of similar size in Michigan and in the United States as a whole, the population in Tecumseh has a slightly higher median level of education, a higher percentage of employed persons in manufacturing industries, and a higher median family income.
>
> The community has little air pollution; levels of solid particulate matter, airborne lead, and carbon monoxide are well below those found in large metropolitan areas. Drinking water, the municipal supply as well

[2]Quoted with permission of the authors and publisher.

as private rural wells, contains high concentrations of calcium, magnesium, and iron and would be classified as "hard" or "very hard" by the usual standards.

Design of the Study and
Research Activities

Detailed descriptions of the design of the study and progress reports have appeared in the literature (116, 120, 128, 130, 131, 246, 270, 356, 357). One of the basic purposes of the investigation is the study of distributions of disease and disability as they exist and develop in a "natural community." Hopefully it will be possible to identify the genetic and environmental factors or constellation of factors which are important in the maintenance of health or the development of disease. The ultimate application of results lies in the field of preventive medicine. Emphasis is on coronary heart disease, diabetes, hypertension, chronic pulmonary disease, and rheumatic disorders, but all diseases and disabilities are of interest.

Field work began in 1957 with the identification of each dwelling unit in the study area and contact with the occupants by trained interviewers (269). Each of the dwelling units is allocated to one of ten samples randomly selected from five strata or geographic areas. "The ten samples are kept current by random allocation of new dwelling units created by construction or conversion. Each cycle of interviewer visits begins with sample I and continues with the other samples in sequence. Dwelling units within each sample are assigned randomly to the interviewers, and each interviewer is assigned a random order of visits. In this way the impact of any bias due to interviewer variability is randomly distributed.

"For analytic purposes all members of the Tecumseh community are identified as individuals, as members of family units, as members of households, and as members of kindreds or bloodlines. They are grouped in sibships as well as in parent-child and husband-wife combinations."(270)

From 1959 to 1960, the first medical examinations of the population were given at the Health Study Clinic, which was located at Herrick Memorial Hospital in Tecumseh. Eight thousand six hundred forty-one persons, representing 88 percent of all persons contacted, were examined. Exhaustive medical histories were first administered by interviewers. The respondents then came to the clinic where physicians from the University of Michigan Medical School administered complete physical examinations except that no rectal or pelvic examinations were given. Laboratory determinations and clinical procedures included the following:

1. Resting electrocardiograms.
2. Pulmonary function including vital capacity (the maximum volume of

air the subject could expire) and $FEV_{1.0}$ (the maximum air expired in one second).
3. Various anthropometric measurements including skinfold thickness.
4. Resting blood pressure.
5. Standard chest X-ray.
6. Blood tests including glucose tolerance, hemoglobin, serum uric acid and rheumatoid factors, and serum total cholesterol.
7. Urine analyses including glucose, protein, acetone, occult blood, and acidity. A microscopic examination was done if albumin was noted.

In the years 1961 to 1965, the second cycle of examinations was conducted in the clinic at Herrick Memorial Hospital. Nine thousand two hundred twenty-six persons, including 2,499 new residents, were examined. This represented approximately 82 percent of persons of all ages living in the defined community. The same general procedures were followed: namely, a complete health history, or updating of the previous one, and an examination at the clinic. Several laboratory tests were added to those included in the first examination. Special hand and cervical X-rays were taken on most of the respondents and special tuberculin and histoplasmin skin sensitivity tests were done on a random 20 percent sample of the population. An exercise step test (to be described later) was given to all medically eligible males and females, age 10 to 69. Habitual physical activity was assessed in males, age 16 to 69, by questionnaire and interview.

A third cycle of examinations was conducted from February 1967 through June 1969. By the time these examinations began, the clinic had been relocated in a separate building. This third cycle of examinations, instead of including all persons resident in the study community, was limited to: (1) persons who had been previously examined at least once earlier, and (2) persons of all ages, whether previously examined or not, who were residing in a 10 percent random sample of dwelling units. Procedures similar to those of the two previous cycles were carried out for all persons in the 10 percent random sample, for all men and women age 35 and older in the community who had been previously examined, and special groups as follows: (a) relatives of all persons identified in the first cycle as having coronary heart disease or diabetes mellitus (case kindreds), (b) relatives of controls without these diseases who are of similar age and sex (control kindreds), and (c) propositi identified as having chronic pulmonary disease, matched controls, and their immediate families. Another pulmonary function test, nitrogen washout, was added; X-rays were limited to a chest film; skin tests for five common inhalant allergens replaced the skin tests of cycle two; a microhematocrit, blood type, and serum triglyceride determinations were added to the blood analyses; and a multilevel treadmill exercise test (to be described later) was given to a sample of the respondents. An abbreviated procedure which did not include a physical examination, chest X-ray, or treadmill test, was employed for all other previously examined persons, age 15 to 34.

In addition to these comprehensive cycles of examinations, studies of less extensive scope were being conducted as outlined in a recent report (270). These ancillary investigations include surveillance of health status between examinations; acute and chronic respiratory disease; dietary assessment; sociological studies; special lipid metabolism study; and environmental studies in which flora and fauna were mapped, atmosphere monitored in several locations, and drinking water analyzed.

2 / Scope of Monograph: Progress, Plans, and Perspectives

Exercise Capacity

The name Tecumseh Community Health Study implies that health is being appraised, when actually there are few, if any, good measures of health. Usually health is defined in a negative way, as freedom from disease. However, one positive way of measuring health is through the determination of an individual's capacity for physical work. Dr. David B. Dill, distinguished exercise physiologist, expressed this point of view a number of years ago (101). When asked what he thought was a good sign of health, Dr. Passmore, a famous Edinburgh physiologist, put it this way: "On my way home my path leads across an open field. There is a bit of a brook and over it a small foot bridge. When I prefer to jump across that stream, I know I'm in good health." (160)

In the first cycle of examinations, no exercise tests were given. However, the second cycle included a simple submaximal step test to estimate work capacity. In the third series of examinations a more sophisticated treadmill exercise was administered to a large percentage of the study population. Some of the respondents in subsequent years will develop coronary heart disease or other disability. It will then be possible to relate the development of disease with measurements of exercise capacity. Considerable time must elapse before a sufficient number of cases are available for this analysis to be of value; hence, these relationships will not be reported at this time. However, the correlation of exercise capacity with various characteristics of the study population have been studied and are discussed in later chapters. Age and sex comparisons and norms for exercise capacity are also included.

In exercise tests it is not only the maximum work output that is important. When an automobile or airplane motor is tested, the evaluation usually is conducted under dynamic conditions. Although defects may not be detected when the motor is idling, when "revved up" it is often possible to detect malfunction or roughness in tuning. For a long time this principle has been applied to the testing of human beings, the hypothesis being that a mild or moderate exercise stress will distinguish finer gradations of fitness of various physiological systems than is possible under resting conditions. The exercise electrocardiogram is an example. In some individuals, abnormalities in the electrocardiogram appear during exercise months or years before the resting electrocardiogram shows any abnormalities. Therefore, exercise tests were included for their possible diagnostic value.

Habitual Physical Activity

The question is frequently raised whether the amount or intensity of physical activity in which one engages is related to the maintenance of health or the development of disease. This notion is not new. Hippocrates, in the fifth century B.C., in his treatise *Airs, Waters, Places*, stated:

> Therefore, on arrival at a town with which he is unfamiliar, a physician should examine its position with respect to the winds and the risings of the sun . . . the mode of life also of the inhabitants that is pleasing to them, whether they are heavy drinkers, taking lunch, and inactive, or athletic, industrious, eating much and drinking little. (320)

In another treatise, *Regimen*, Hippocrates advocated exercise as preventive medicine:

> Exercise should be many and of all kinds; running on the double track increased gradually; wrestling after being oiled, begun with light exercises and gradually made long; sharp walks after exercises, short walks in the sun after dinner; many walks in the early morning, quiet to begin with, increasing till they are violent and then gently finishing. (177)

Ramazzini, an epidemiologist who wrote what is probably the first book on occupational diseases more than 250 years ago, believed a sedentary life contributed to ill health.

> All sedentary workers, tailors above all and women who do needlework in their homes day and night to make a living, suffer from the itch, are a bad color, and in poor condition. . . . These workers, then, suffer from general ill-health and an excessive accumulation of unwholesome humors caused by their sedentary life; this applies especially to cobblers and tailors. (300)

With the increase in use of labor-saving devices and motorized transportation, the role of sedentary living as a factor in disease susceptibility has assumed greater significance. This is particularly true in recent years— degenerative diseases now appear more frequently as causes of death. Considerably less progress has been achieved in preventing these conditions, which are more closely correlated with habits of living, than in preventing or curing certain childhood diseases and acute infections.

The most direct approach in studying the effects of regular exercise on disease susceptibility is an experimental investigation in which sedentary people embark on an exercise program. Then, after a certain amount of time has passed, it can be ascertained how many people died from or have developed a particular disease. In fact, Karvonen (194) quotes the famous English physician, Heberden, who wrote in 1802 about heart disease as follows: "I know one who set himself a task of sawing wood half an hour every day, and was nearly cured." This classical approach, if carried out with proper controls, should provide a clear answer to the question of whether a leisure-time exercise program provides protection against coronary heart disease. It was the author's pleasure to serve for about three years on a committee, organized by Dr. Samuel M. Fox and Dr. Henry L. Taylor under the aegis of the U.S. Public Health Service, to evaluate the feasibility of such an intervention study. An estimate of the number of subjects necessary to undertake an investigation of this kind will have a sobering effect and can dampen one's enthusiasm for this approach. Remington and Schork (306) have calculated these estimates. Let us assume the annual incidence of coronary heart disease in sedentary middle-aged men in the United States to be about 1 percent, not an unreasonable estimate (117). If we assume (a) that a program of exercise would reduce this incidence by about 25 percent, (b) that 10 percent of the men would discontinue the exercise program each year,[1] and (c) that reasonable assumptions are made about the statistical techniques, then we would need to begin with a sample of 12,000 men in the experimental group and 12,000 control subjects, and the experiment would have to continue for five years to detect a significant effect of exercise on coronary heart disease. This is not an impossible task, but a formidable one indeed!

Using high-risk subjects would help somewhat but would not eliminate the need for very large numbers of subjects. One could exercise people who have already developed heart disease, but this is not quite the same problem.

Some species of animals, because of their short life span, can be used for experimental research on cardiovascular disease. Heart disease has been produced in many kinds of animals, but the applicability of results to human beings is always questionable. Furthermore, with regard to physical exercise,

[1]This is an optimistic figure. The dropout rate would be considerably higher (353).

applications require the specification of duration, frequency, and intensity of exercise, and such quantification cannot be obtained in animal studies.

Clearly other approaches are needed. One kind of investigation, called a retroactive study, involves the identification of individuals who have developed a disease or died as a result of it. Next, an attempt is made to ascertain how physically active these people were before disease or death occurred. The simplest way is to determine their occupation. These studies are relatively inexpensive because records of death and even disease are fairly accessible, at least in highly developed countries. These investigations are efficient in that it is not necessary to have a large population under surveillance with the expectation that only a small percentage of the people will develop a particular disease. As a case in point, Kraus and Raab (208, pp. 96–97) list seventeen studies in which death rates from heart disease were related to habits of physical exercise (mostly occupational). In all but one, the death rate was higher among the sedentary subjects.

The picture is impressive until it is recognized that these studies do not represent seventeen different approaches. Instead, one study has been repeated a number of times. This is not meant as a criticism; it is obviously important to confirm results before one can place much confidence in them. Nevertheless, the same limitations apply in varying degrees to all these investigations. An excellent discussion of problems associated with retrospective or cross-sectional studies of this kind may be found in a report by Taylor and colleagues (354). Briefly, the most important limitations include the following:

1. Selection of an occupation (and hence the amount of habitual physical activity) may have been determined, at least in part, by the subject's state of health. Men whose health is impaired may gravitate to the less strenuous occupations. In most of the studies quoted by Kraus and Raab, serial determinations of the subject's occupation and state of health are not available, hence the influence of job selection or changes in occupation cannot be assessed.
2. The effects of physical activity may be indirect and may only operate through some other factor, for example, body fatness. The apparent association may even be incidental. It is conceivable, for example, that sedentary occupations are psychologically more stressful and the stress may be the significant factor, not the lack of physical activity. A comprehensive assessment of the subjects and their environment is usually not available in retrospective studies, so the independent effects of physical activity cannot be separated from other possible biological or social factors.
3. The measurement of habitual physical activity is crude, ordinarily restricted to assumptions about a kind of occupation. Leisure-time physical activity has rarely been estimated, and yet, in the lives of many people, a significant amount of physical activity can only be obtained during off-job hours.

In prospective investigations such as the Tecumseh Community Health Study, it should be possible to overcome these difficulties, at least to a considerable extent. The effects of selection or change in occupation or in leisure-time physical activity may be assessed because data were collected earlier in life when there was no sign of ill health. Second, because a host of other measurements are available on the subjects as well as measurements of the physical and social environment, the independent effects of physical activity may be appraised. Finally, more accurate estimates of physical activity are possible because it is not necessary to rely upon a job classification alone. Because serial observations are available, changes in habitual physical activity may be related to changes in other measurements.

The deaths in the Tecumseh population, even from coronary heart disease, have been too few to provide meaningful data, as yet, for definitive prospective analysis. However, laboratory measures known to be associated with certain diseases (so-called risk factors) have been studied in relation to habitual occupational and leisure-time physical activity. It has also been possible to eliminate the effects of other factors on these relationships. The results will be reported in subsequent chapters.

Strength and Physical Fitness

Arm and grip strength was measured in most of the respondents during the second series of examinations in Tecumseh, and these measurements together with others may provide information about body build, or at least provide a means to identify the mesomorphic (muscular) type. However, the analysis of these data is not complete and, for the most part, will not be included in this monograph.

A battery of physical fitness tests was administered to virtually all children in grades four through twelve in the Tecumseh population. Of course, very few of these children have been identified as having any disease. However, it may some day be possible to determine whether or not the kind of physical fitness measured by such tests has any predictive value for health or disease in later life. Meanwhile it is possible in this monograph to report relationships between physical fitness and certain disease risk factors.

Population Comparisons

Virtually the entire population of Tecumseh, Michigan, and its immediate surrounding area are under study. It has thus been possible to select certain groups and compare them to the rest of the population. In later chapters, comparisons in various measurements will be made between the healthy and sick, athletes and nonathletes, and children enrolled in physical education and those not enrolled. The Tecumseh population is a natural living group of unselected, mostly healthy, people. Data on this group provide an excellent backdrop for comparing other outside populations. One such comparison, between business executives and age-matched Tecumseh subjects, will be reported in this monograph.

Familial Relationships

Ultimately it will be possible to investigate exercise capacity, habitual physical activity, strength, and physical fitness within families. Fathers and mothers can be compared with each other and with their children. Siblings may be compared. However, these analyses are left for the future.

Previous Publications

Most of the data reported herein have been published in greater detail in highly technical journals. References to these sources are provided. The purpose of the present monograph is to bring this material together in one place summarized in somewhat nontechnical language, and to include a review of related literature.

Chapter 3

Occupational and Leisure-Time Physical Activity

Method of Assessment

Methods for determining energy cost (i.e., oxygen consumption) of various activities have been available for many years. These determinations in the field, by indirect calorimetry, require the subject to wear a mask or nose- and mouthpiece, and to breathe into Douglas bags or other apparatus. The gas exhaled must be carefully measured and the concentration of oxygen and carbon dioxide in a sample determined. The development of accurate electronic methods of measuring gas concentrations has simplified the method, but it is still a time-consuming procedure. Furthermore, in assessing the habitual activity of people, serious additional problems are encountered. Occupational and leisure-time activities vary greatly throughout any given day, from day to day, and from season to season. This requires extensive sampling throughout the year with each individual. Additionally, the psychological impact and the physical problems of measuring energy expenditure introduces an artificiality which may result in nonrepresentative data.

As discussed elsewhere (240), some investigators have used heart rate, ventilation, or respiratory rate as an estimate of strenuousness of activity. In the laboratory, on any given day in a particular individual, these parameters are fairly closely related to energy cost. However, during occupational or leisure activity the physiological measurements may be influenced by factors other than energy expenditure. In some investigations, pedometers[1] have been used, but with this technique, work done with the upper body is not measured. Furthermore, pedometer, heart rate, and ventilation data, although easier to obtain, are subject to the same practical limitations as the direct measurement of energy expenditure.

In epidemiologic investigations of essentially healthy people in which the development of disease is to be studied, large populations are needed. The methods referred to in the preceding paragraphs are not useful in such studies. Most investigators have had to utilize questionnaires and/or interviews to estimate energy expenditure, despite the problems and inaccuracies associated with this approach.

Although individual investigators have devised questionnaires or interviews for their own use, the methods have rarely been critically analyzed. Also, the interpretation of activity recall records has generally been subjective. In most studies, only occupational work was considered because it is less difficult to estimate the energy cost of occupational tasks than leisure-time activities. When the physical activity forms utilized in recent epidemiologic research are examined, it is found that few attempt to assess the energy requirements of both occupation and leisure, and none attempt to objectively quantify the ratings of physical activity.

Method Used in Tecumseh

A preliminary attempt was made in Tecumseh to assess the physical activity by a *self-administered* form. This was a revision of a questionnaire used in an earlier study (370). The first 10 percent probability sample of dwelling units in Tecumseh provided about 350 men and women for this investigation (269). Despite field trials of preliminary forms and numerous revisions in the wording of questions, there was still considerable evidence of misinterpretation by the respondents. Many questions were unanswered or answered incompletely. It was concluded that in a total population containing people of varying occupations and education, a personal interview was necessary to increase the accuracy. It was also concluded that accurate estimations of the length of time women spent in household tasks was not possible utilizing these forms; therefore, the assessment of physical activity of women has not been attempted in Tecumseh. Questionnaire and interview forms were again revised and field-tested. A second revision followed which was used on the final 80 percent of the male population during the second cycle of examinations (1962 to 1965). This form was published (304) and was used in the second and third series of examinations with all males 16 years and older in Tecumseh who were not in school.

The interviewer, at first contact, delivered a self-administered questionnaire to the respondent. If the respondent was not employed at the time,

[1]An instrument attached to the leg which purports to measure distance walked.

a modified form was used. In the questionnaire, inquiries were made about occupation(s), hours worked, transportation to and from work, and the time and effort expended on home repairs and maintenance. Leisure-time sports, gardening, and other physical activities were checked on a list.

At next contact, the trained interviewer spent from thirty minutes to an hour with each respondent inquiring about the physical activity involved in the respondent's occupation and leisure activities. A prepared supplementary interview form was used for occupation(s) and for *each* leisure-time activity checked. The questionnaire and interview forms were designed to estimate physical activity during the preceding year. Physical activity during the preceding three months was also recorded, but this proved to be of no additional value.

The supplements were designed to probe for differences in intensity of physical activity. For example, it was learned in preliminary work that the occupational title was frequently of little or no value in estimating the physical activity associated with the job. Therefore, questions were asked to determine as accurately as possible how much actual physical activity was involved. In only one general occupation, farming, was this not possible. Therefore, the interviewer ascertained that the man actually worked on a farm and was not a "gentleman farmer." She also determined approximately how many hours a week the respondent worked on the farm. It is clear that another questionnaire is needed to assess specifically the physical activity of farmers. Until such a form is used in the Tecumseh population, these workers will be treated as a special group.

Questions about leisure-time activities were designed to estimate strenuousness of activities. For example, it was determined whether a man fished while sitting in a boat or walking in a stream, because the energy costs are quite different in these two methods of fishing. Similarly, if a respondent plays baseball on an organized team, he likely expends more energy than in playing "catch" with his young son. It is important from the standpoint of energy cost to make such distinctions.

Objective Scoring

It has not been possible as yet to establish the validity of our procedures by employing an external criterion such as direct assessment of energy cost, recording the heart rate, or making direct observations. However, it was recognized that an objective system had to be developed for interpreting and scoring these data. Therefore, the reliability of interpretation of the record was studied as follows: Two randomly selected samples from the data collected, each composed of twenty completed questionnaire and interview forms, were subjectively ranked by three judges independently with the most active respondent at the top and the least active at the bottom.

This was done for each of three components, namely: occupation, leisure, and occupation plus leisure. After approximately six weeks (sufficient time for the first ranking to be forgotten), each judge ranked the two samples a second time. The rank order correlations illustrating each judge's consistency in ranking within sets ranged from 0.96 to 0.99. Because the two rankings by each judge within each sample correlated so highly, the first ranking was arbitrarily selected for the comparisons *between* judges. The correlations between judges for both samples ranged from 0.90 to 0.99 for occupation, from 0.66 to 0.82 for leisure, and from 0.86 to 0.94 for occupation plus leisure. The mean of the three judges' subjective ranks for each respondent was then calculated for occupation, leisure, and occupation plus leisure. This was done for both samples. These mean ranks formed the criterion for the development of an objective scoring system. A simple objective system was desirable to enable clerks to score the record with little subjective judgment.

The first step in the preparation of the scoring system was the construction of a table of metabolic costs for various occupational and leisure tasks. These have been published (304) in the form of ratios of work metabolism to basal metabolism (WMR/BMR). This expression, employed earlier by Dill (100), eliminates the necessity of considering the subject's body weight, converting the work to calories, etc. The method assumes that a task performed by a heavy person raises his metabolism to the same extent percentagewise as the same task performed by a person weighing less, even though the caloric expenditure might be different. Because much of the activity involves moving one's own body weight, errors in making this assumption probably are not serious. There are other limitations to the scoring procedure. The occupational and leisure activities are those found in this particular area. Data on energy cost of many activities are available in the literature, so reasonably good estimates could be made. However, for other activities data are lacking, and, therefore, our estimates may not be accurate. It is also well known that the energy cost for the same task varies from individual to individual depending upon skill, walking surface, equipment, clothing, environmental conditions, terrain, and perhaps other factors. Finally, the activities themselves are carried out in a different manner in various parts of the world, and even within areas of the United States. Hence, this table may have to be amended and/or changed when applied to another population or another culture. We are not deluded into thinking this scoring system provides precise quantitative values. Therefore, the average metabolic cost of occupational and/or leisure tasks as calculated is used to classify people into one of three physical activity categories.

The procedure to categorize subjects was as follows. The work-to-basal ratio (WMR/BMR) for a particular activity was multiplied by the number of hours during the year in which the subject engaged in that activity. This was repeated for all activities requiring appreciable energy expenditure.

The products were summed and divided by the total hours, to arrive at a weighted average work-to-basal metabolic ratio. When estimating the overall activity, the leisure and occupational activities were averaged, weighted, of course, by the hours in each. For this purpose several assumptions were made. Because it was not feasible to determine how many hours each subject slept or how many hours were involved in eating meals, shaving, etc., it was assumed that each respondent slept eight hours a day, at a work-to-basal ratio of 1. When the subject was not sleeping or doing physical work, it was assumed he was eating, reading, driving a car, watching television, or engaging in other quiet activities. An average work-to-basal metabolic ratio of 1.8 was assigned to the time spent in this way.

In order to assess the validity of this objective method of calculating the average energy expenditure, the subjective ranking of the two sets of twenty respondents was used as a criterion. The subjects were then ranked by average expenditure according to the objective method just described. Table 3.1 gives the rank order correlation coefficients for the comparison of the two sets of twenty respondents each. It is clear that the two methods give approximately the same results.

Table 3.1

RANK ORDER CORRELATION COEFFICIENTS COMPARING RANKS BASED ON OBJECTIVE SCORING SYSTEM WITH AVERAGE SUBJECTIVE RANK

	Set 1 $(N = 20)$	Set 2 $(N = 20)$
Occupation only	0.97	0.90
Leisure only	0.90	0.91
Occupation and leisure	0.86	0.87

Reproduced from (304) with permission of the publisher.

Classification by Habitual Physical Activity

The next step was to reduce the various energy cost estimates to indices which might be used to classify participants in the study. The various indices calculated for each of the 1,929 males interviewed were as follows:

A. *Occupation*
   1. The average number of hours per week of occupational work including all occupations of the respondent.
   2. A weighted mean work-to-basal ratio utilizing the WMR/BMR associated with each of the subject's occupational activities, weighted by the number of hours spent at each. This reflects the average *rate* of energy expended on the job.
B. *Leisure*
   3. The average number of hours per week in which the respondent was

engaged in *active* leisure. This does not include hours reading, playing cards, etc.

4. A weighted mean work-to-basal ratio similar to number 2 above but for active leisure. This mean reflects the average *rate* of energy for the active leisure, not the *total* energy expenditure during active leisure.

5. A leisure index which is the sum of each active leisure pursuit (WMR/BMR × hours spent). This reflects the total energy expenditure during active leisure.

C. *Occupation and Leisure*

6. A weighted mean work-to-basal ratio as in number 2 including both occupational and leisure activities. This index reflects the average 24-hour daily rate of energy expenditure.

A weighted standard deviation of the individual work-to-basal ratios was calculated. This was done for occupation and leisure activity separately, and for occupation and leisure combined. A coefficient of variation (ratio of the standard deviation WMR/BMR to the mean WMR/BMR) for each individual was also calculated for occupation, leisure, and occupation and leisure. These six indices reflect the variation in physical demands experienced by an individual. However, for many individuals there was only one energy estimate for his occupation or leisure. Therefore, after studying the distributions of these six indices and their correlations with the other indices, their interpretation was difficult or impossible; hence they were not used.

As one might expect, occupational work-to-basal ratio (i.e., an estimate of average rate of energy expenditure on the job) was highly correlated with the work-to-basal ratio based on both occupational and leisure-time activities.[2] In dealing with the entire population of men, it is clear that the leisure-time component adds little information to the determination of physical activity on the basis of occupation alone. This is so because the time spent at work, eight hours per day in many subjects, accounts for the greatest part of the total activity calories.

Leisure time, however, may be of value if one intends to discriminate within homogeneous groups, such as office workers. In a group of about 300 executives studied (125, 249), almost all had very sedentary occupations. The only significant differences in energy expenditure were to be found in leisure activities.

Next, the respondents were grouped by decade of age. Distributions for each of the six indices and for each of the age groups were examined. The plan was to classify respondents who were in the lowest 20 percent (for a particular index in a particular age group) as least active, the middle 60 percent as intermediate, and the upper 20 percent as most active. In most

[2]The correlation coefficients between mean work-to-basal ratio for occupation (No. 2) and for occupation and leisure (No. 6) ranged from 0.80 to 0.90 among the ten-year age groups.

instances this was possible. However, in the case of hours worked (number 1 above), about half of the respondents were placed in the lower group, about 30 percent in the middle group, and about 20 percent in the upper group. For each index, the proportions in each group (lower, middle, and upper) were the same for all age categories.

Habitual Physical Activity and Age[3]

Physical activity data were obtained from males age 16 through 69 who were not in school. Many of the subjects between 16 and 22 years of age were full-time students, hence the small number of subjects under 20 were included with the 20 to 29-year-olds. For purposes of the physical activity-age-occupation analyses, males who were unemployed were excluded. Farmers were included only in the tabulations of leisure-time activities.

Occupational Physical Activity

Figure 3.1 (left side) discloses that both the hours worked per week and the strenuousness of the work decreased slightly with age. This is not unexpected. The other occupational activity indices showed similar trends. The slight decrease in hours worked per week with age is explained mainly by a decrease in hours worked by subjects in managerial occupations (Figure 3.2, upper graph), whereas the decrease with age in mean rate of energy expenditure on the job is due mainly to a decrease in the service and labor occupations (Figure 3.3). It is not surprising that the decrease in occupational activity with age is not greater. Many occupations are very sedentary and it is hardly possible as one becomes older to reduce the energy expenditure further. Additionally, there are many men in the unskilled, semiskilled, and skilled occupations who have worked in these occupations all their lives. In some cases it would be difficult to change to a less strenuous occupation later in life. Although these age effects are not great, they are statistically significant, and necessitated studying habitual physical activity within age groups.

Leisure-Time Physical Activity

Tecumseh, Michigan, is situated close to many recreational facilities. Within the city are located five tennis courts, ten bowling lanes, three swimming pools (including one heated year-round pool and a 5-acre pond in a 22-acre park). A recreation center has space available for dance,

---

[3]Information on habitual physical activity in this monograph is based upon data from the second cycle of examinations. Much of the data on age and habitual physical activity was published in greater detail elsewhere (87, 88, 89).

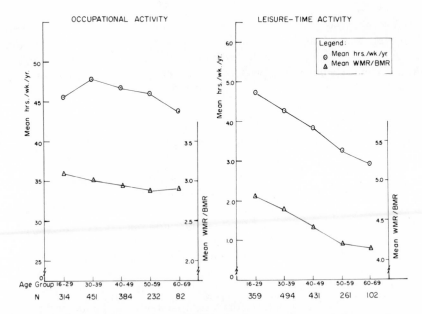

Fig. 3.1 Left panel: mean hours worked and mean estimated energy expenditure (WMR/BMR) in occupation. Right panel: mean hours and mean estimated energy expenditure during active leisure pursuits.

exercise, and instructional groups. Local schools are used for various city activities, including exercise groups and a judo club. Softball leagues are open to all men in the city. Within a 20-minute drive from Tecumseh there is a large recreation area which includes lakes suitable for swimming, boating, and fishing in the summer, and hills for winter skiing. The lands surrounding Tecumseh can be used for small game and bird hunting.

The length of time available for participation in any leisure activity is usually governed by season, which varies in length for each activity. In order that the time during which the respondents participate in leisure activities be comparable for all activities and that it be additive to occupational values for other analyses, the number of participation hours was recorded as hours per week prorated for the year preceding the interview. The degree of involvement would, therefore, be recorded as number of hrs/wk/yr.

Disregarding age, the percent participation in the various leisure activities for at least 30 minutes per week on the average is shown in Table 3.2. The decrease with age in hours spent in active leisure activities can be seen in Figure 3.1. In Figure 3.4 subjects were placed into one of three groups on the basis of the most active leisure activities (highest WMR/BMR) in which the subjects participated for at least 1.5 hrs/wk/yr, for all leisure activities combined. Very few persons participated regularly (at least 1.5 hrs/wk/yr) in leisure activities requiring a high level of energy expenditure; i.e.,

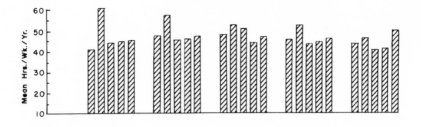

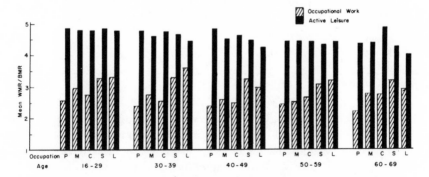

Fig. 3.2 A comparison of the mean number of hours per week per year spent during occupational work and active leisure activity among occupational groups (ages 16 to 69). The occupational groups are: P—professional and technical, M—managerial, C—clerical and sales, S—skilled and semi-skilled, and L—service and labor. Reproduced from (89) with permission of the publisher.

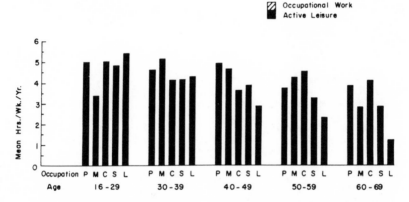

Fig. 3.3 A comparison of the mean weighted mean work-to-basal ratios during occupational work and active leisure activity among occupational groups (ages 16–69). The occupational groups are: P—professional and technical, M—managerial, C—clerical and sales, S—skilled and semi-skilled, and L—service and labor. Reproduced from (89) with permission of the publisher.

Table 3.2

PERCENT PARTICIPATION FOR ACTIVE LEISURE-TIME ACTIVITIES

Activity	*Percent Participation for All Ages and Occupations ($N = 1648$) (0.5 Hrs per Wk per Yr)*
Lawn-mowing with power mower	40
Garden work	29
Hunting	25
Fishing from boat, shore, or ice	23
Walking (3 mph)	19
Home improvement	18
Bowling	13
Golf	12
Swimming (can swim 50 ft)	8
Social dancing	8
Conditioning exercises	8
Softball or baseball (game play)	4
Softball or baseball (non-game play)	4
Table tennis	3
Lawn-mowing with ride mower	3
Basketball (non-game play)	2
Ice skating or roller skating	2
Badminton	2
Square dancing	2
Hand mowing	2
Archery (target)	2
Tennis	1
Water-skiing	1
Stream fishing, wading	1
Archery (hunting)	1
Bicycling (12 mph)	1
Canoeing or rowing (for pleasure)	1
Basketball (game play)	0
Canoeing or rowing (in competition)	0
Handball or squash	0
Snow-skiing	0
Volleyball	0
Swimming (cannot swim 50 ft)	0
Sailing	0

WMR/BMR of at least 8. Only 3 percent of males age 16 to 29 were in this group. Participation was 1 percent or less in the older age groups. The majority of persons participated for at least 1.5 hrs/wk/yr in activities requiring an energy expenditure of 4.0 to 7.9 times the basal level.

The ten most popular active leisure activities in which the respondents participated are shown in Figure 3.5. Percentage of participation for each activity is shown for each age group. A more detailed analysis is given in reference 88.

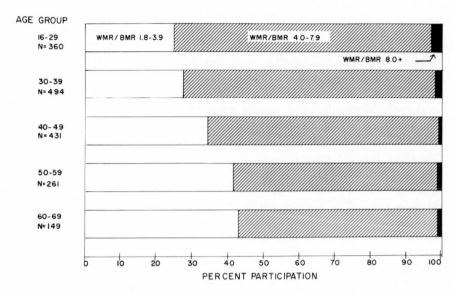

Fig. 3.4   Relation of age to participation, at least 1.5 hours per week, in leisure activities of various energy costs.

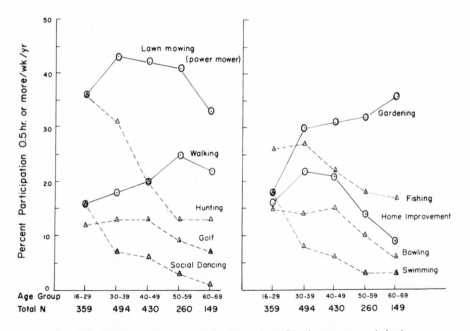

Fig. 3.5   Relation of age to participation, at least 30 minutes per week, in the ten most popular leisure-time activities.

Excluded from Figure 3.5 are all the leisure activities in which very few people participated. The criteria were arbitrarily selected to exclude any activity in which only 5 percent or less of the total population participated for a minimum of 0.1 hr/wk/yr. Those activities not included are lawn-mowing with a hand mower, archery, fishing while wading, basketball (game), volleyball, handball, squash, sailing, canoeing or rowing for pleasure, canoeing or rowing in competition, snow-skiing, and lawn-mowing with a ride mower. The WMR/BMR's of many of these activities were higher than the more popular activities.

There is, in general, a decrease in participation in leisure activities with increased age. In most cases this decrease is statistically significant. However, in the case of walking, no change was observed between the younger and older age groups, and in the case of garden work the age groups 30 and older were significantly more involved with this activity than the 16 to 29 age group. Three activities, lawn-mowing, golf, and home improvement, had a slight increase in participation in the 30 to 39 age range compared to the 16 to 29 age range. This was followed by a decrease in participation to age 69. It appears that the decrease in participation with increased age is reflected in all activities (gardening and walking excluded), but the decrease is somewhat greater in the more strenuous activities.

The correlation coefficients between age groups for the rank-ordering of the leisure activities are presented in Table 3.3. In this table only the coeffi-

Table 3.3

RANK ORDER CORRELATION COEFFICIENTS BETWEEN
AGE GROUPS FOR 0.1 HR/WK/YR MINIMUM
PARTICIPATION IN ACTIVE LEISURE ACTIVITIES

Age	30–39	40–49	50–59	60–69
16–29	.936[a]	.915	.882	.662
30–39		.953	.874	.736
40–49			.907	.795
50–59				.877

[a]*The higher the correlation coefficient, the more closely were the various leisure activities related with respect to percentage of participation.*
Reproduced from (88) with permission of the publisher.

cients for a minimum participation of 0.1 hr/wk/yr or more are reported; however, the other minimum hours of activity have similar correlations. There was little change from one age group to the next age group in the rank of activities in which subjects participate. The greatest changes between any two adjacent age groups occurred between those subjects in the 50 to 59 age group and those in the 60 to 69 age group. A fairly high correlation was observed between the type of activities in which subjects age 16 to 29 participated through to subjects age 50 to 59. These results support those of earlier investigations (15, 381).

Zborowski (381) studied the effect of aging upon the recreational life of a group of men and women over 50 years of age who provided information with regard to their recreational activities at the age of 40 and at their present age. He found that the patterns of activity established at the age of 40 tended to persist into later years. Baley (15) studied trends in habits of recreational activity. Subjects were grouped into age classes of 20 to 29, 30 to 39, 40 to 49, and 50 to 59 years. He found, as was observed in the present study, that with respect to frequency of participation, the majority of the recreational activities maintained their *rank* among the various age groups but older men participated less frequently in almost all forms of recreational activity.

Occupation and Habitual Physical Activity[4]

The respondents were classified by occupation held at the time of interview using the census occupation codes. Occupational classifications used in this study were: Professional and technical (000–195),[5] Managerial (250–285, R), Clerical and sales (301–360, Y, Z, 380–395, S), Skilled and semiskilled (401–555, Q, 601–721, T, W), and Service and labor (810–890, P, 960–973, X).

The average number of hours spent on the job in the various occupations in different age groups is shown in Figure 3.2. During occupation work the mean hours ranged from 40 to 60 hrs/wk/yr. As mentioned earlier, the hours spent at work changed very little across age groups. A notable exception can be seen in the managerial group; those in the younger age group spent a good deal more time at work than those in the older age groups.

The mean rates of energy expenditure at occupational work and at active leisure are shown in Figure 3.3. In all ages, the blue-collar workers were engaged in activities during work which required a higher rate of energy expenditure than the activities of the white-collar workers. These differences between the rates of energy expenditure of the blue- and white-collar workers were statistically significant ($p < .05$) at ages 30 to 59. This would be expected almost by definition of the occupation.

The hours spent at active leisure generally decreased across ages 16 to 69 in most occupational groups (Figure 3.2). The greatest decreases in

---

[4]Additional details are available in several publications (87, 89).

[5]Numbers in parentheses refer to the codes for occupations found in U.S. Bureau of the Census, 1960 Census of Population, Alphabetical Index of Occupations and Industries (rev. ed.), U.S. Government Printing Office, Washington, D.C., 1960.

active leisure time, ages 16 to 59, were observed in the blue-collar workers (skilled and semiskilled, and service and labor). The white-collar occupations (professional and technical, managerial, and clerical and sales) changed very little in the number of hours spent at active leisure between ages 16 and 59. All occupations showed a decrease in time spent at active leisure in the oldest group (60 to 69).

The differences in the mean rate of energy expenditure during leisure among the occupational groups was not striking. Because it was not possible to determine how much physical activity was involved in farm tasks, the farmers were excluded from the analyses concerned with occupational work. However, the active leisure pursuits of the farmers were studied. In ages 16 to 69 they spent fewer hours in active leisure than most other occupational groups, and except for age 30 to 39, the rate of energy expenditure at active leisure was also lower.

The eight specific active leisure activities in which 12 percent or more subjects participated for a minimum of 0.5 hours per week per year were analyzed in more detail by occupation. The results are reported in Table 3.4. With the exception of golf, few statistically significant relationships were observed between occupation and participation in leisure activities, and these were scattered randomly throughout the various age groups. In golf the differences were significant at two age groups (30 to 39 and 40 to 49) and for the total of all ages. The professional and technical occupations had the highest percent participation in golf in the younger ages (16 to 39). In age group 40 to 49, the three white-collar occupations (professional and technical, managerial, and clerical and sales) had higher percent participation in this sport than did the blue-collar occupations (skilled and semiskilled, service and labor, and farmers). After age 50 the professional and technical and clerical and sales groups decreased in participation slightly and the managerial group contained the most golf participants. Other significant relationships for the total of all ages were observed for "Fishing from Boat, Shore, or Ice," "Bowling," and "Leisure Walking." Farmers participate to a lesser extent in all three of these activities.

Two major factors must be noted that may limit the extent to which the results of this study may be generalized beyond the study area. The focus of this study was on active leisure; the sedentary forms of leisure were excluded. In addition, the data were collected in one community; therefore, the results may not be applicable to other areas that are very different in geographical location and sociological structure.

Clarke (67) found systematic differences between the frequency of participation in certain types of leisure activities and levels of occupational prestige. He found a curvilinear relationship between golf participation and occupational prestige. The middle prestige group was the most active in golf. He felt that golf represented a good example of how an activity was

Table 3.4

PERCENT PARTICIPATION IN ACTIVE LEISURE ACTIVITIES
BY AGE AND OCCUPATION
(PARTICIPATION 0.5 HRS OR MORE PER WK PER YR)

Age (Yrs)	Occupation*						Age (Yrs)	Occupation*					
	P	M	C	S	L	F		P	M	C	S	L	F
Lawn-Mowing with Power Mower							*Garden Work*						
16–29	43	50	31	35	26	43	16–29**	25	19	11	16	13	36
30–39	46	54	39	41	50	37	30–39	25	26	44	28	31	47
40–49	43	38	45	47	27	26	40–49**	20	28	14	37	29	24
50–59**	41	43	58	45	43	7	50–59	29	31	32	38	23	21
60–69	45	27	14	35	0	58	60–69	30	24	71	38	20	40
Total	44	44	39	42	32	33	Total	24	27	27	30	22	34
Hunting							*Fishing from Boat, Shore, or Ice*						
16–29	19	42	41	35	39	40	16–29	32	32	22	27	35	15
30–39	24	31	22	36	19	33	30–39	25	34	25	29	31	14
40–49	21	23	10	20	7	22	40–49	18	26	14	25	20	11
50–59	14	17	5	13	15	17	50–59	24	14	32	17	14	14
60–69	9	18	14	16	0	10	60–69	0	14	14	22	20	15
Total	20	26	24	27	23	27	Total**	22	26	23	25	27	14
Walking							*Home Improvement*						
16–29	25	8	30	14	16	11	16–29	13	14	14	18	21	7
30–39	23	17	11	18	31	12	30–39	23	25	26	21	20	19
40–49	27	17	5	23	20	9	40–49	21	30	18	22	14	11
50–59	29	22	42	23	43	10	50–59	15	13	19	13	7	19
60–69	10	18	29	19	20	20	60–69	22	5	14	11	0	6
Total**	25	17	22	19	25	11	Total	20	21	18	19	16	13
Bowling							*Golf*						
16–29	11	8	22	17	6	13	16–29	36	12	18	9	16	2
30–39	14	20	17	14	19	5	30–39**	25	26	19	8	6	0
40–49	16	20	23	13	20	6	40–49**	32	27	32	6	0	0
50–59	14	26	16	7	0	0	50–59	14	26	16	7	9	0
60–69	0	5	0	8	20	5	60–69	9	27	0	5	0	0
Total**	13	18	19	13	11	6	Total**	27	24	20	7	7	1

*Occupation: P—Professional and Technical; M—Managerial; C—Clerical and Sales; S—Skilled and Semiskilled; L—Service and Labor; F—Farmers.
**Differences between the observed and expected frequencies of participation were significant (p < .05).
Despite the Chi Square values, differences between the observed and expected frequencies were not considered significant if more than 2 expected frequencies of participation for any of the 6 occupation groups were less than 5, or any expected frequency was less than 1 (72).
Reproduced from (87) with permission of the publisher.

being transformed from the exclusive pastime of a few wealthy individuals to a popular activity for many people. In the past, golf may have been restricted to the wealthy members of society. Today, however, many opportunities exist for almost anyone to participate in golf at a moderate cost. The blue-collar worker is developing some interest in this activity. If social mobility increases in the next few years, more blue-collar workers may become interested in this activity and the relationship between golf participation and occupation may disappear.

Other investigations (67, 106, 190, 201, 305, 348, 372, 381) have reported that socioeconomic status and the extent and type of leisure activities in which their subjects participated were related. In many of these studies (67, 106, 201, 372, 381) educational attainment or family income was used as a measure of social status, whereas job classification was used in the present study. In addition, three of the previous studies (67, 305, 372) were conducted almost two decades ago. Since then rapid social changes may have occurred which obliterate earlier class-related participation (191).

Havighurst (161), in a study of free-time activity, found that there was much variability in leisure activity among people of a given sex, age, or social class. Leisure habits were observed to depend more upon personality than age, sex, or social class. Dowell (106), in a very recent study, used occupation to classify workers into social groups. He found wide differences between occupational groups in the types of recreational activities in which they participate. Dowell studied all forms of leisure activities; whereas in the present study only active leisure activities were studied.

Summary

The present study has described the active leisure activities of males in a total community, Tecumseh, Michigan. In addition, the relationship of occupation and age with participation in the most popular activities has been analyzed. These findings have practical significance for the planning of leisure services by both public and private agencies. The leisure activities in which people are involved change little with age. However, the time spent decreases with age. This reflects, at least in part, that interest and skills in active sports and recreation are most often learned when young. It is not that older people cannot learn new skills, but they seem to lack the time and/or inclination to do so. This evidence also indicates that the skills and interests in activities suitable for older people should be developed in school-age children.

Because this study shows little relationship between occupation and leisure activities, the prevailing occupations in an area might be less important in planning curricula in physical education than might have previously been thought. Perhaps the most surprising observation is the low participation rate in almost all active leisure-time activities.

Chapter 4 / Physiological Response to Exercise: Step Test

A simple submaximal exercise in the form of a step test was administered to most of the respondents, age 10 to 69, in Tecumseh during the second series of examinations. A more sophisticated step test, treadmill, or bicycle ergometer exercise would have been preferable, but the facilities, equipment, or personnel were not available for a more elaborate assessment of work capacity.

Submaximal exercise tests, in which heart rate is measured during or after the exercise, have a long history. The development of the Harvard Step Test (43) did much to popularize this simple approach. The theoretical bases, applications, limitations, and modifications of the Harvard Step Test have been reviewed elsewhere (239). Very briefly, the test rests on the observation that if a person is physically active or conditioned for strenuous work, his heart rate during and after a standard *submaximal* exercise will be lower than the heart rate of an unconditioned (untrained) person living a sedentary life. Although the complete explanation for this is not clear, most work physiologists believe the lower heart rate is due, at least in part, to the fact that a person used to vigorous exercise has a greater cardiac stroke volume (amount of blood pumped with each beat of the heart), both at rest and during exercise, than the less active person. The heart rate during and after a standard exercise is very sensitive to a conditioning program, decreasing after a few weeks or months of training, and increasing again soon after training is terminated. Nevertheless, the heart rate response to exercise is not a good predictor of work performance (endurance)

29

or metabolic capacity—i.e., the maximum oxygen that an individual can take in from the air and use in the tissues during exercise (239). Doubtlessly this is partially because of other factors that may affect the heart rate, the most important being high ambient temperature and emotions. High temperature, particularly with high humidity, raises the heart rate because one of the important functions of circulation, besides delivering oxygen to the tissues and removing waste products, is the maintenance of body temperature. Fortunately, temperature was controlled in Tecumseh so this was not a confounding variable. The effect of the test conditions on emotions and hence on the heart rate is not known. It is generally accepted, however, that this factor becomes less important as the exercise becomes more strenuous.

Method

The submaximal test used in Tecumseh was a modification of the Harvard Step Test. The subjects were required to step onto an 8-inch bench at the rate of 24 steps (4-count sequences) per minute for 3 minutes. This is a rate of energy expenditure roughly equivalent to five times the basal metabolic rate (23). The electrocardiogram, from which heart rate was measured, was recorded with the subject sitting before the exercise, during the exercise, and for 5 minutes after the test while the subject was again sitting.

The subjects usually came to the clinic in family groups in the afternoon, early evening, or on Saturday morning. They were not necessarily in a postabsorptive state. All tests were administered in an air-conditioned laboratory (72 to 76° F.).

Subjects

The test was administered to males and females, age 10 to 69 years, who were not excluded for medical reasons. Pregnant women were excluded. There were thus 6,497 respondents, age 10 to 69, who were participating in the overall study. Approximately 84 percent (5,448) were given the exercise test. The remaining 16 percent were excluded because of pregnancy, for various medical reasons, and in a few instances because the air-conditioning system failed. The medical exclusions comprised mainly respondents with a history or symptoms of heart disease or stroke, acute and severe respiratory infections, severe arthritis, hypertension (systolic > 170 and/or diastolic > 110), and various orthopedic disabilities.

The number of subjects in the study, by each age group, is shown in Table 4.1. This table also contains the number and percentage of respondents who took the step test, and the number and percentage who were unable to complete the test, or who for some reason did not perform the test properly. The data on which this report is based include only data on the subjects who performed the exercise properly.

Sex and Age Comparisons[1]

The mean pre-exercise, terminal (i.e., 3-min) exercise, and 1-min post-exercise heart rates are shown in Figures 4.1, 4.2, and 4.3, respectively. It has long been known that resting heart rates are higher in females throughout the age range (173). It is clear from Figure 4.1 that our data show much the same picture. There is a greater difference between males and females in exercise and post-exercise heart rates (Figures 4.2 and 4.3) than in pre-exercise heart rate. This also has been shown previously for a limited age

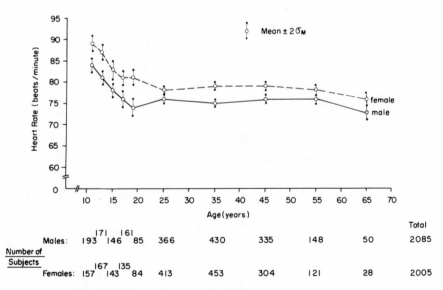

Fig. 4.1 Mean sitting pre-exercise heart rates in males and females. Reproduced from (255) with permission of the publisher.

[1]A more detailed analysis may be found in two references (255, 256).

Table 4.1   NUMBER AND PERCENT OF SUBJECTS TAKING STEP TEST

| | Age Groups | | | | | |
	10–19	20–29	30–39	40–49	50–59	60–69
MALES						
Total N in study	998	478	622	542	329	192
Test not done properly or stopped	5(0.5)[a]	8(1.7)	17(2.7)	15(2.8)	17(5.2)	6(3.1)
Did not take test	34(3.4)	22(4.6)	55(8.8)	101(18.6)	122(37.1)	63(32.8)
Completed test properly	959(96.1)	448(93.7)	550(88.5)	426(78.6)	190(57.8)	123(64.1)
Completed test, HR data obtained	756[b]	336	430	335	148	50
FEMALES						
Total N in study	936	597	702	555	337	209
Test not done properly or stopped	8(0.8)	10(1.7)	20(2.8)	31(5.6)	33(.98)	14(6.7)
Did not take test	61(6.5)	74(12.4)	97(13.8)	118(21.3)	143(42.4)	159(76.1)
Completed test properly	867(92.7)	513(85.9)	583(83.4)	406(73.1)	161(47.8)	36(17.2)
Completed test, HR data obtained	686	413	453	304	121	28

[a] Percentages are in parentheses. The denominator for calculating these percentages in each case is the total males (or females) in the study in the particular age group.

[b] The numbers in this line and the last line of the table correspond to the numbers in Figures 4.1–4.3. Through a misunderstanding, ECGs were not recorded after 2 min 30 sec of the exercise in about 23 percent of the subjects even though they completed the test properly. The total population had been divided into ten. 10 percent random samples. The subjects in each sample were examined before the next sample was scheduled for the clinic. The misunderstanding was not discovered until about the first 23 percent of the subjects had been tested. Because these were essentially randomly selected, it is unlikely that any bias resulted.

Reproduced from (256) with permission of the publisher.

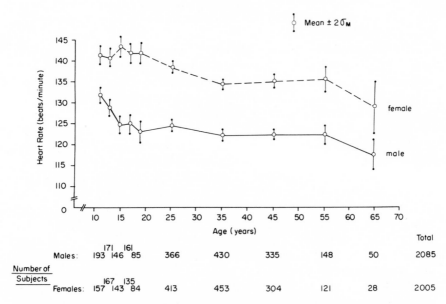

Fig. 4.2 Mean heart rates at end of 3-minute exercise in males and females. Reproduced from (255) with permission of the publisher.

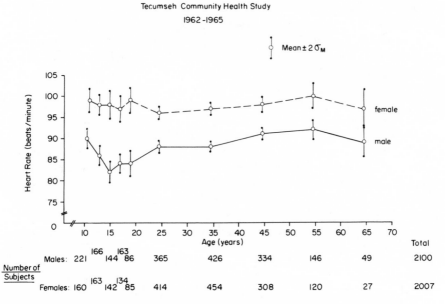

Fig. 4.3 Mean sitting heart rates 1 minute after exercise in males and females. Reproduced from (255) with permission of the publisher.

group (11, 14, 235). The higher heart rates in females are likely related to lower hemoglobin concentration (288) and perhaps a smaller relative heart size (382) and less difference in the oxygen content of the arterial and venous blood (A-V difference) in females (66).

The pre-exercise heart rate in the young children (age 10 to 11) averaged about 84 beats per minute in males and 88 beats per minute in females and decreased to about 75 by age 20 in males and 79 at age 20 in females (Figure 4.1). Our observations of higher resting heart rate in children and little change with age during adult life are similar to Robinson's data (314) and his summary of the literature. The relatively high pre-exercise heart rates in our subjects probably reflect an increase in anticipation of the exercise. The reason for the lower heart rates in the oldest subjects is not clear.

The observations of Robinson (314), Åstrand (9), and Henschel (164) are similar to ours; namely, little difference among various adult age groups in heart rate at the end of a submaximal exercise (Figure 4.2). On the other hand, Norris and collaborators (276) reported a positive age–heart rate relationship in submaximal work of a lower intensity than that employed by us. Rhyming (308) showed a correlation of age with heart rate response in a submaximal exercise of greater intensity.

In Figure 4.3 it can be seen that the post-exercise heart rates increase from about age 15 through age 55 or 60. In order to study the relationship between age and recovery heart rate with the effect of terminal heart rate eliminated, data on all male subjects whose heart rate at the end of exercise (terminal heart rate) was 120–124 beats per minute were studied separately. Their recovery heart rates were plotted by age in Figure 4.4 (left panel). The significant increase in recovery heart rates with age is striking, especially at 30 sec post-exercise. It is still evident at later post-exercise periods, but as recovery proceeds the age trend becomes less noticeable. Recovery heart rates of male subjects whose terminal heart rate was 130–134 and 140–144 were analyzed in the same way. These data are graphed in the center and right panels of Figure 4.4. Similar results were observed in female subjects.

Several authors (109, 276, 314) reported delayed recovery of heart rate *after* submaximal exercise in older people. In the Durnin and Mikulici study (109), the age effect was not statistically significant. It is generally accepted that the maximum heart rate during exhaustive exercise is decreased with age (9, 11, 314, 332). The observed delayed recovery could be because in older people the terminal heart rate in submaximal exercise is closer to the maximum heart rate in these subjects. For example, in a young man of age 25, the average terminal heart rate (Figure 4.2) of 125 represents only about 65 percent of his maximum of 193 beats per minute (314). On the other hand, this same terminal heart rate in a man age 50 represents 72 percent of his maximum and in a man age 65 it would renresent 75 percent

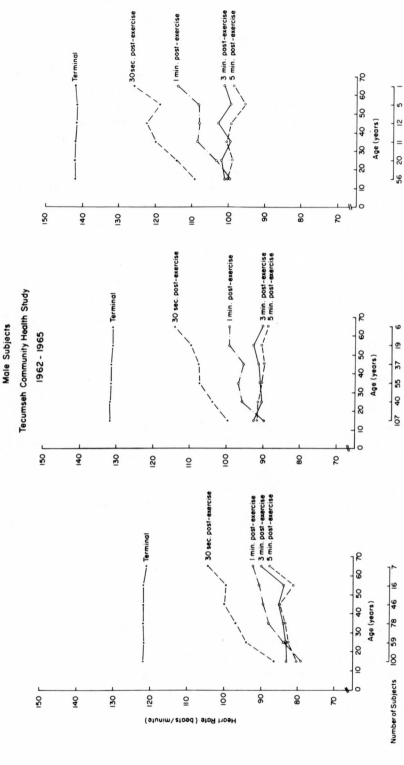

Fig. 4.4 Age curves for post-exercise heart rates in subjects with about the same terminal exercise heart rate (males). Reproduced from (256) with permission of the publisher.

35

of maximum. In our older respondents, the terminal heart rate is about the same as in younger persons and yet these older individuals appear to be utilizing more of their reserve and depending more upon anaerobic metabolism. Support for this concept can be found in the observation by Baldwin and co-workers (14) that oxygen consumption of older men remains elevated longer during recovery from exercise than in young men. This is also supported by Berg (20). Furthermore, Robinson (314) reported greater reduction in alkaline reserve in old than in young subjects following submaximal exercise, which likely reflects greater blood lactate accumulation.

One may postulate that the older subjects might be heavier, and hence doing more physical work, to explain the higher post-exercise heart rates. If body weight or body fatness were a significant factor, one would expect the terminal exercise heart rate to show a relationship to age. This was not true (Figure 4.2). Furthermore, although mean body weight in this population increased somewhat in females from age 35 to 60, this was not the case in males (247). In a sample of our population, age 20 to 69 (248 males, 143 females), there was no correlation of body weight or height with either the terminal or the one-minute post-exercise heart rate. Previous studies in adults have also indicated little or no correlation between heart rate following a standard step test and body weight, height, lower extremity length, lean body mass, or percent lean body mass (239).

Perhaps, as Simonson (332) has postulated, following studies of the effect of exercise on the flicker fusion frequency, there is decreased excitability of the central nervous system in older subjects. This might explain why the terminal heart rate of older respondents is no higher even though there is increased anaerobic metabolism. However, none of these explanations rule out the possibility of greater peripheral pooling of blood during recovery as being partially responsible for the delayed heart rate recovery following exercise. Changes with age in muscle fibers that might restrict gas exchange in the tissues have been pointed out (235).

Percentile Norms

Within any age group heart rate during and after exercise are closely correlated. As an example, the correlation coefficients for the 30 to 39-year age group are shown in Table 4.2. Other age groups show similar results. Hence, for comparing individuals it makes little difference which heart rate period is used. In Tables 4.3 and 4.4, percentile ranks are given for males and females. The heart beats were counted on the electrocardiogram from 30 seconds after exercise to 1 minute after exercise.

Table 4.2

CORRELATION COEFFICIENT MATRIX OF HEART RATES DURING AND
AFTER STEP TEST FOR SUBJECTS AGE 30–39[a]

	Ex., 2 min 30 sec		Ex. (terminal), 3 min		Post-ex., 30 sec		Post-ex., 1 min		Post-ex., 2 min		Post-ex., 3 min		Post-ex., 5 min	
	M	F	M	F	M	F	M	F	M	F	M	F	M	F
1. Ex., 2 min 30 sec	—	—	.91	.95	.83	.80	.79	.79	.77	.73	.74	.72	.77	.71
2. Ex. (terminal), 3 min	.91	.95	—	—	.83	.83	.78	.81	.75	.75	.73	.73	.74	.72
3. Post-ex., 30 sec	.83	.80	.83	.83	—	—	.90	.91	.86	.86	.82	.84	.83	.82
4. Post-ex., 1 min	.79	.79	.78	.81	.90	.91	—	—	.89	.91	.86	.88	.86	.86
5. Post-ex., 2 min	.76	.73	.75	.75	.86	.86	.89	.91	—	—	.89	.91	.89	.90
6. Post-ex., 3 min	.74	.72	.73	.73	.82	.84	.86	.88	.89	.91	—	—	.90	.92
7. Post-ex., 5 min	.77	.71	.75	.72	.83	.82	.86	.86	.89	.90	.90	.92	—	—

[a]*Number of subjects ranged from 400 to 585 for females and from 424 to 542 for males.*

Reproduced from (255) with permission of the publisher.

Table 4.3

HEART BEATS FROM 30 SECONDS TO 1 MINUTE AFTER A STANDARD 3-MINUTE STEP TEST, 8-INCH BENCH, 24 STEPS PER MINUTE: MALES ONLY (30-SECOND COUNT)

Percentile	Age															Precentile
	10	11	12	13	14	15	16	17	18	19	20–29	30–39	40–49	50–59	60–69	
95	37	36	35	34	32	32	31	34	33	34	34	35	37	37	35	95
90	39	38	39	36	33	34	34	35	34	36	36	38	39	40	37	90
85	40	39	40	37	35	35	36	37	36	38	38	40	41	42	39	85
80	42	40	41	38	36	36	37	38	37	40	40	41	42	43	41	80
75	43	41	42	39	37	37	38	40	38	41	41	42	44	44	43	75
70	44	41	43	40	38	38	39	41	39	42	42	43	44	45	44	70
65	45	42	43	41	39	39	40	42	40	43	43	44	45	46	45	65
60	46	43	44	42	40	40	41	43	41	44	44	45	46	47	46	60
55	46	44	44	43	41	41	41	43	42	45	45	45	47	47	47	55
50	47	45	45	44	42	42	42	44	43	46	46	46	48	48	48	50
45	48	46	46	45	43	43	43	45	43	47	47	47	49	49	49	45
40	49	47	47	46	44	43	44	46	44	48	48	48	50	50	50	40
35	50	48	47	47	45	44	45	47	45	48	49	49	50	51	50	35
30	51	49	48	48	46	45	46	49	46	49	50	50	52	52	51	30
25	52	50	49	49	47	46	47	50	48	50	51	51	53	53	52	25
20	54	52	51	50	48	47	48	51	49	52	53	52	54	55	53	20
15	56	54	52	52	50	48	50	53	50	53	54	54	55	56	55	15
10	58	56	55	54	52	50	53	55	53	55	56	56	57	58	56	10
5	61	60	59	56	56	53	57	57	57	57	59	59	60	62	59	5
Number of Subjects	89	89	81	67	61	67	85	61	41	33	334	389	310	136	41	

Table 4.4

HEART BEATS FROM 30 SECONDS TO 1 MINUTE AFTER A STANDARD 3-MINUTE STEP TEST, 8-INCH BENCH, 24 STEPS PER MINUTE: FEMALES ONLY (30-SECOND COUNT)

Percentile	10	11	12	13	14	15	16	17	18	19	20-29	30-39	40-49	50-59	60-69	Percentile
95	39	38	39	40	40	36	38	37	36	45	39	39	41	41	42	95
90	42	40	40	42	42	39	42	40	41	47	42	42	43	44	43	90
85	44	42	42	44	44	42	44	42	45	48	43	43	44	46	44	85
80	46	44	43	46	45	44	45	44	47	49	45	45	45	47	45	80
75	48	45	44	47	46	45	47	45	49	50	45	46	46	48	46	75
70	49	47	46	48	47	47	48	46	51	50	46	47	47	49	47	70
65	50	48	47	49	48	49	49	47	52	51	47	48	48	50	48	65
60	51	49	48	50	49	50	50	48	53	51	48	49	49	51	49	60
55	52	50	49	51	50	52	51	50	53	52	49	50	50	52	50	55
50	54	51	50	52	51	53	52	51	54	52	50	51	51	53	50	50
45	55	52	51	53	52	54	54	52	54	53	52	52	52	54	51	45
40	56	54	52	54	53	56	55	53	55	54	53	53	54	55	52	40
35	57	55	53	55	54	57	56	54	56	54	54	54	55	56	53	35
30	58	56	54	56	55	58	58	56	56	55	55	55	56	57	54	30
25	60	57	56	57	56	60	59	57	57	56	56	56	57	58	55	25
20	61	59	57	59	58	62	61	59	58	57	58	57	59	59	57	20
15	63	61	59	62	60	64	63	61	59	58	60	59	61	61	58	15
10	65	63	62	64	62	67	65	63	61	60	62	62	63	63	60	10
5	67	67	65	69	65	70	67	66	64	62	66	66	67	66	63	5
Number of Subjects	68	84	90	61	65	62	69	51	35	42	380	420	276	106	24	

Chapter **5 / Physiological Response to Exercise: Treadmill Test**

Although oxygen uptake capacity is being measured in many laboratories throughout the world, such studies generally involve volunteers and/or small numbers of subjects who may be tested repeatedly. The requirements of the Tecumseh study, as is true of many large epidemiologic investigations, dictate that the administration of the exercise tests must be feasible with subjects who are unfamiliar with work capacity tests. In Tecumseh, the test also had to be suitable for a wide age range, 10 to 69 years, and both sexes. The safety of the subjects had to be insured even though the test was not administered in a hospital setting. It was, therefore, necessary to evaluate and modify laboratory methods for use in a large-scale investigation. Because other investigators have shown interest in measuring metabolic capacity in epidemiologic studies, our experiences and protocol have been described (90, 245).

Method

It is preferable to gradually increase the severity or strenuousness of an exercise test. When testing subjects who vary greatly in age and metabolic capacity, a fixed work test will be too strenuous for some and will understress others. Tests of increasing strenuousness (sometimes called multistage tests) have generally utilized a bicycle ergometer, a motor-driven treadmill,

40

and more recently, a variable height bench for stepping. A treadmill was selected for our study for several reasons. It is relatively safe; in a step test when the height of the bench or rate of stepping is increased, it is not uncommon for older subjects to trip. Mechanical efficiency is essentially the same over a wide age range and for conditioned and nonconditioned subjects. The rate of work can be controlled and the subject must maintain the rate to stay on the mill. In the United States, unlike many other countries, riding a bicycle is not a common activity for adults. However, most people do at least some walking every day, hence little training on the treadmill is needed. Also, no seat or other adjustments are necessary as is true in the case of the bicycle ergometer.

The test employed by us consists of walking on the treadmill at 3.0 miles per hour at zero grade for 3 minutes; thereafter, the mill is raised 3 percent every 3 minutes with speed maintained. In subjects over 59 years of age, the speed is maintained at 2.0 miles per hour. The percent grade is calculated as the height over the belt travel (sine of the angle), not the rise over the run (tangent of the angle) as defined in engineering terms. The sine of the angle is frequently used in physiological studies. The Balke test (17) is an example.

The energy cost for a 70-kg man walking 3 mph is roughly 5 calories per minute (1 liter of O_2 uptake). This is approximately three times the resting rate. Raising the treadmill 3 percent increases the oxygen uptake for a man of this size by about 250 milliliters per minute. The subject continues to walk until he is exhausted except as noted below. After a demonstration by the technician of the correct method of walking without holding on to the handrails, the subject practices for about a minute at 2 mph. Then the speed is increased to 3 mph. Completely naive subjects up to the age of 60 are able to walk easily and in a relaxed manner following this much practice. Although most subjects from 60 to 69 could walk at this rate, we prefer to have all subjects in this age group walk at 2 mph. The grade change schedule is the same as with younger subjects.

Several procedures were automated for greater accuracy and to save technician time. A programmer was constructed so that once the test is started, the treadmill would automatically elevate 3 percent every third minute. A sound signal was built into the circuit to warn the technicians that the final (third) minute of a particular level is approaching. This enabled them to prepare for taking certain measurements. At precisely two minutes at each level (i.e., the start of the third minute) a signal appeared on the record. Another mark indicated the end of the third minute at a particular treadmill grade. This enabled the technician to make measurements on the record during precisely the last minute of a work load.

Physiological Parameters

During the exercise test, the physiological variables described below were monitored on an oscilloscope and recorded on an eight-channel photographic recorder. The ECG signal is transmitted from the multichannel recorder into a single-channel electrocardiograph, where a tracing can be recorded at any time by the attending physician. This is done because some physicians prefer to see the ECG recorded at a paper speed and on an instrument with which they are familiar. During most of the test, the multi-channel paper speed is 2.5 mm/sec with 1-sec time lines. However, at pre-scribed intervals before, during, and after the exercise, the paper speed is 50 mm/sec with 0.04-sec time lines. This faster speed is used to facilitate ECG interpretations (see Figure 5.1).

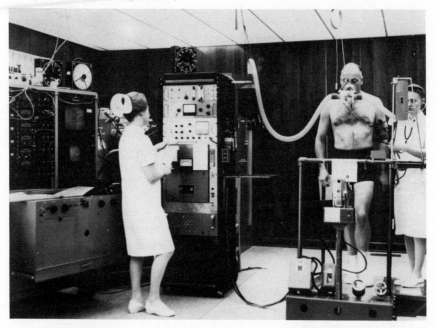

Fig. 5.1 Subject walking on the treadmill while various physiological measure-ments are being recorded.

Electrocardiogram

Plastic electrodes with a well to hold the electrode paste are used. Shielded wires connect the subject via a ceiling cable to the recorder. A bipolar lead system recommended by Blackburn and colleagues (30) as being more sensitive to abnormalities than other single leads is employed. This requires that the reference electrode be placed on the *manubrium sterni* and the exploring electrode at the chest position V_5 (CM_5). The ECG can be monitored at sweep speeds up to 200 mm/sec on the oscilloscope independently of the paper recording speed.

Heart Rate

A cardiotachometer which reads the heart rate from two successive R or S spikes of the ECG provides a visual display of the beat-by-beat heart rate and also was recorded on paper (Figure 5.2).

Blood Pressure

This is recorded manually with a sphygmomanometer by a technician before the exercise, at each grade during the exercise, and at specific intervals during the recovery period. Fifth-phase diastolic is used although sphygmomanometer diastolic blood pressure during exercise is known to be inaccurate in some instances (164).

Ventilation

The recommendations of Dill (99) have been especially helpful in developing our procedures. For measuring ventilation, a dry gas meter (Model D-4 or CD-4, Parkinson-Cowan Measurement Company) was used on the intake side. These are excellent inexpensive meters which measure minute ventilation up to 160 liters or more with no appreciable error. The accuracy of these meters has been reported elsewhere (90). The CD-4 model is slightly more accurate and more suitable than the D-4 model. A potentiometer was installed to follow the needle of the meter. This adds no appreciable resistance. The output of the potentiometer is linear and is recorded on one channel of the multichannel recorder. Each time the subject inhales, the excursion of the needle is recorded and thus respiration rate, tidal volume, and minute ventilation can be readily measured (Figure 5.2). A Triple-J breathing value which enabled the subject to breathe with no noticeable resistance even during heavy work was employed.

Oxygen Uptake

In order to measure oxygen uptake, it is necessary to determine the concentration of oxygen, carbon dioxide, and nitrogen in the exhaled air as well as the ventilation. Of course, it is necessary to determine only two of the gases, the third being determined by subtraction. The most accurate method for doing this is by means of chemical gas analyzers, but the time required for their use is prohibitive in large epidemiologic studies. In recent years, electronic analyzers have been developed to give rapid, in-line concentrations of the gases. We have studied the accuracy of the analyzers using the chemical analysis as a standard (90, 245). The results indicated that the percent oxygen and carbon dioxide in the exhaled air can be accurately

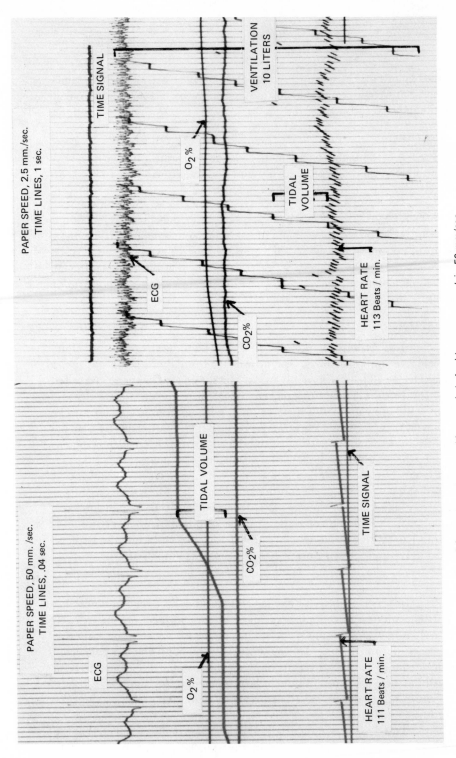

Fig. 5.2 Typical photographic record. Left side, paper speed is 50 mm/sec. Right side, paper speed is 2.5 mm/sec. Reproduced from (245), *Amer. J. Epidemiol.*, 91 (1970), 41, with permission of the publisher.

measured by a paramagnetic oxygen analyzer and capnograph, respectively. In using the electronic meters, three test gases with various known percentages of oxygen, carbon dioxide, and nitrogen concentrations (determined by Scholander analysis) were employed for calibration before each subject was tested. The concentrations of O_2 and CO_2 as measured electronically, together with ventilation, corrected to standard conditions, were then substituted in the well-known equation (73) for calculating oxygen uptake:

$$\dot{V}_{O_2} \text{ consumed} = \text{Vol air inspired} \times \frac{20.93}{100} - \text{vol air expired}$$
$$\times \frac{\%O_2 \text{ in expired air}}{100}$$

These oxygen uptakes were compared with oxygen uptake as calculated from the gas concentrations measured by the micro-Scholander chemical analyzer (Table 5.1). Agreement is remarkably good. What is especially interesting is the fact that if only oxygen concentration is measured and nitrogen percentage in the exhaled air is assumed to be 79.04 (i.e., respiratory exchange ratio assumed to be 1.00), the oxygen uptake can be estimated quite accurately. This is not surprising in view of the discussion by Otis (282). From his calculations, even with the respiratory exchange ratio ranging from 0.7 to 1.3, the maximum error to be expected would only be 6.3 percent. This has important implications for epidemiologic research because it means oxygen uptake capacity may be estimated fairly accurately with a minimum of equipment, namely an oxygen analyzer and a dry gas meter. It is necessary also to construct a mixing chamber containing baffles to obtain a mixed expiratory sample which is then directed to the gas analyzers. The 6-liter and 12-liter mixing chambers used were patterned after the one described by Dill (99).

It should be pointed out that the data for making the comparisons in Table 5.1 were collected by technicians during routine testing of subjects in the Tecumseh Community Health Study. These data were collected in the course of the investigation to maintain quality control on the data. In practice, one sample of respiratory gas generally was taken daily and analyzed on the Scholander apparatus for comparison with the electronic analyzer values. In Table 5.1, of the 109 measurements, 19 were maximal oxygen uptake measurements and these are shown separately.

Computer Program

A computer program was developed[1] to avoid the routine calculation of oxygen uptake and related measures. Precoded sheets were pre-

[1]Mr. Jacob Keller wrote the program for the IBM 360 computer.

Table 5.1

COMPARISON OF OXYGEN UPTAKE VALUES MEASURED BY SCHOLANDER CHEMICAL ANALYZER WITH VALUES MEASURED BY ELECTRONIC ANALYZERS

	Scholander	O_2 *and* CO_2 *Analyzers in Combination*	*r*	*SE of Est.*
Oxygen uptake (l/min), total sample N = 109				
Mean*	1.996	1.996	0.998	0.049
SD	0.73	0.73		
Oxygen uptake (ml/kg body wt/min), total sample, N = 109				
Mean	28.42	28.36	0.996	0.856
SD	10.21	10.20		
Maximal oxygen uptake (l/min) N = 19				
Mean	3.022	3.032	0.990	0.066
SD	0.44	0.45		
Maximal oxygen uptake (ml/kg body wt/min), N = 19				
Mean	42.79	42.95	0.990	0.918
SD	6.27	6.44		

*Difference between the mean for the oxygen uptake calculated by the Scholander chemical analyzer and the means for the oxygen uptake calculated by the electronic meters were not significant ($p < .05$).

Reproduced from (245), *Amer. J. Epidemiol.*, 91 (1970), 43, with permission of the publisher.

pared which required only the entry of data by the technician. Data on each of these precoded sheets was transferred to IBM cards. The computer plots the test gases and interprets, from the linear regression, the actual percent ages of gases in the respiratory sample at each grade level. The computer then calculates oxygen uptake, respiratory exchange ratio, oxygen pulse, etc., for each grade level and prints the information as illustrated in Figure 5.3. Finally, the computer plots, for each exercise grade level, the oxygen uptake in liters per minute as the ordinate and heart rate as the abscissa. An example is shown in Figure 5.4. The oxygen uptake–heart rate plot was scrutinized for each subject as a check for errors. If any points appeared to be out of line, the basic data were checked by the technician to see if a measuring or transcription error was made. Each week the data for the subjects tested were punched and sent to the computer. Within a week or two the printouts were back in the laboratory to be studied. Two technicians could readily test one subject per hour with good quality control over the data.

Reproducibility

In order to investigate the reliability of the treadmill test, 27 male subjects were asked to come back to the clinic a second time, generally within two weeks. There were 10 subjects selected at random in the age group 10

ID 00898, AGE 38, EXAM DATE 20-02-68   LENGTH OF TEST - 22 MINUTES

LEVEL	GRADE	V O2 L/MIN	V O2 ML/KG/MIN	V CC2	VE L	F	VT	R	O2 PULSE ML/BEAT	V EQ L/V O2	W KGM/MIN	V O2 ML/KGM	WT KG	FH B/MIN	BPS MMHG	BPD MMHG	RFS
00	0	.37	5	.33	10.7	14	.8	.88	4.4	28.78	0	.00	79	86	130	090	0
01	0	1.32	17	.97	24.4	17	1.4	.73	12.6	18.74		.00	79	105	150	080	0
02	3	1.42	18	1.28	28.2	17	1.7	.90	12.4	19.96	191	7.44	79	114	152	070	0
03	6	1.58	20	1.45	31.8	18	1.8	.92	13.1	20.18	381	4.15	79	121	142	090	0
04	9	1.81	23	1.71	36.2	19	1.9	.94	13.5	20.01	572	3.17	79	134	150	080	0
05	12	2.23	28	2.13	45.3	23	2.0	.95	14.7	20.34	763	2.93	79	152	160	080	0
06	15	2.60	33	2.72	60.4	27	2.2	1.05	15.6	23.16	953	2.72	79	167	162	070	0
07	18	3.01	38	3.32	78.3	32	2.4	1.10	16.5	25.90	1144	2.63	79	182	172	070	0
08	21	3.09	39	3.44	84.4	36	2.3	1.11	16.7	27.18	1335	2.32	79	185	170	060	0
09	0	9.99	9999	9.99	999.9	99	99.9	9.99	99.9	99.99	0	9.99	79	165	182	072	0
10	0	9.99	9999	9.99	999.9	99	99.9	9.99	99.9	99.99	0	9.99	79	128	170	080	0
11	0	9.99	9999	9.99	999.9	99	99.9	9.99	99.9	99.99	0	9.99	79	118	160	080	0
12	0	9.99	9999	9.99	999.9	99	99.9	9.99	99.9	99.99	0	9.99	79	113	140	080	0
13	0	9.99	9999	9.99	999.9	99	99.9	9.99	99.9	99.99	0	9.99	79	111	130	070	0
14	0	9.99	9999	9.99	999.9	99	99.9	9.99	99.9	99.99	0	9.99	79	112	122	080	0
15	0	9.99	9999	9.99	999.9	99	99.9	9.99	99.9	99.99	0	9.99	79	110	120	062	0

Fig. 5.3 Computer printout of observations and calculations of interest. The first column refers to sample; i.e., 00 is taken when subject is sitting, 01 walking at 0% grade, etc. Col. 2, grade in percent. Col. 3, oxygen uptake in liters per min. Col. 4, oxygen uptake in liters per kg body wt. Col. 5, CO_2 production in liters/min. Col. 6, ventilation in liters/min. Col. 7, frequency of respiration. Col. 8, tidal volume in liters. Col. 9, respiratory exchange ratio. Col. 10, oxygen uptake per heart beat in ml. Col. 11, ventilatory equivalent in liters of ventilation per liter oxygen uptake. Col. 12, vertical work in kilogram-meters. Col. 13, oxygen uptake in ml per kilogram-meter of vertical work. Col. 14, body weight in kg. Col. 15, heart rate. Col. 16, systolic blood pressure. Col. 17, diastolic blood pressure (5th phase). Col. 18, coded reason for stopping exercise. 999 indicates no data. Reproduced from (245), *Amer. J. Epidemiol.*, 91 (1970), 44, with permission of the publisher.

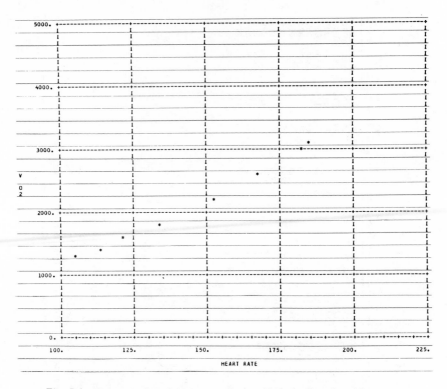

Fig. 5.4 Computer plot of oxygen uptake in ml/min (ordinate) and heart rate (abscissa). Computer has been programmed to plot only heart rate above 99/min. Reproduced from (245), *Amer. J. Epidemiol.,* 91 (1970), 44, with permission of the publisher.

to 19, 9 in age group 30 to 39, and 8 in age group 50 to 59. Figure 5.5 contains a comparison of the two tests in exercise time, maximal heart rate reached, oxygen uptake at a heart rate of 150, and maximal oxygen uptake. In the 50 to 59 age group, maximal oxygen uptake was estimated by extrapolating from the individual oxygen uptake–heart rate curve (Figure 5.4 is an example) up to a heart rate of 165.

Criteria for Stopping Exercise

Criteria for stopping the exercise were discussed in detail and agreed upon before the exercise testing was initiated. These are enumerated below. A physician was present whenever the subject was over 25 years of age and the physician signed the log book and entered pertinent comments at the end of the test.

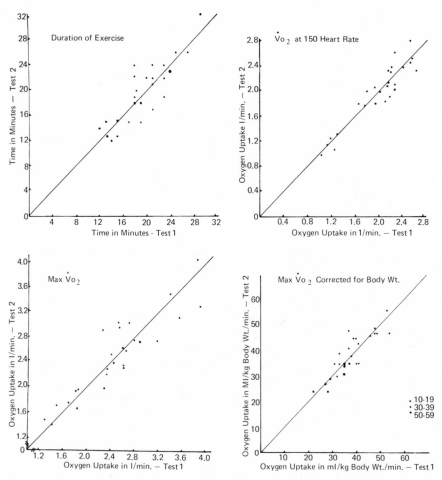

Fig. 5.5 Reproducibility of the treadmill test. A. Exercise time. B. Maximal heart rate reached by the subject. C. Oxygen uptake at a heart rate of 150 beats per minute. D. Maximal oxygen uptake. Reproduced from (245), *Amer. J. Epidemiol.,* 91 (1970), 45, with permission of the publisher.

Specific Indications for Stopping Exercise

1. Symptoms
    Chest pain suggestive of angina
    Claudication
    Severe dyspnoea
    Extreme fatigue
    Dizziness or faintness
    Marked apprehension, mental confusion, or lack of coordination
2. Signs
    a. Physical signs
    Staggering

Pallor

Cyanosis

b. Electrocardiographic signs

Frequent VPSs, one or more approximately every 10 beats

Ventricular paroxysmal tachycardia or atrial paroxysmal tachycardia

Second- or third-degree heart block

Complete bundle branch block, left, right, or indeterminate

Symmetrical T-wave inversion, 3 mm or more deep, not present in pre-exercise standing ECGs, in persons age 30 years or over ST-segment depressions 2 mm or more with horizontal or downward slope of ST-segment, elevations of 2 mm or more

If any of these signs were present, a 12-lead electrocardiogram was taken before the subject left the clinic.

If the exercise was not terminated for one of the above reasons, the endpoint of exercise was the subject's own estimate of exhaustion, if he was 10 to 39 years of age. For subjects 40 to 59 years of age, the test was terminated when the heart rate reached 160. For subjects 60 to 69 years of age, the test was terminated at a heart rate of 150. In the older age groups (40 to 69), if the subject felt exhausted and could not continue the exercise, the test was terminated even though the specified heart rate had not been reached.

The attending physician, laboratory supervisors, and technicians had been instructed in emergency procedures should these have been necessary. They included mouth-to-mouth resuscitation and external cardiac massage. A defibrillator, cardiac synchronizer, and appropriate drugs were maintained in the state of readiness in the laboratory. During the two and one-half years, about 1,400 subjects, age 10 to 69, were tested on the treadmill as described with no untoward effects and no need for the emergency procedures.

Subjects

In Chapter 1 it was pointed out that the round-three physical examinations and standard laboratory tests were given to (a) all men and women, age 35 and over, who had been examined previously, (b) relatives of special groups described in Chapter 1, even though they were under age 35, and (c) all residents of a 10 percent sample of dwelling units in the study area. Inasmuch as about an hour was required for each treadmill test, it was possible to give this test to only about a third of the subjects who came to the clinic. The decision was arbitrarily made to confine the exercise test to all medically eligible males age 35 to 69; males 10 to 34 in the special groups, (b) above; and males and females age 10 to 69 in the 10 percent sample in (c) above. At the time the respondent came to the clinic for the physical examination, those medically eligible were scheduled for the exercise test on another day, usually within a week. Tables 5.2 and 5.3 show the populations involved and the number who were actually given the exercise test.

Medical exclusions included those people with heart disease, arthritic or other orthopedic disabilities which interfered with walking, hypertension, and a variety of less frequently encountered conditions. Pregnant women were excluded. The largest group to be excluded were those with cardiovascular disease. The exclusion criteria for these cases is shown below.

Criteria for Exclusion from Exercise Tests

All respondents in the Tecumseh project are given a medical examination, as well as a standard 12-lead electrocardiogram, before being scheduled for the exercise test. Using the following criteria,[2] the respondents are either scheduled for the exercise test or excluded from it.

1. History of myocardial infarction; probable or suspect.
2. History of angina pectoris; probable or suspect. Note that all histories in which chest pain was reported must be screened by a physician prior to scheduling for exercise tests.
3. Congestive heart failure, probable or suspect, by history or physical examination.
4. Medication: digitalis, quinidine, nitrates, or other vasodilating drugs.
5. Electrocardiographic criteria: the following Minnesota codes (2) call for exclusion from exercise tests: I 1, 2, 3; IV 1, 2; V 1, 2, 4; VII 1, 2, 4; VIII 2, 3, 4, 5. In addition, any electrocardiogram which is not in any of the above categories but is clinically suggestive of myocardial infarction calls for exclusion; this requires that all electrocardiograms *must* be screened after the first clinic visit, and that any subjects who show these abnormalities must not be scheduled for the exercise test.
6. Murmurs: any diastolic murmur, any systolic murmurs thought to be due to mitral insufficiency, aortic stenosis, septal defect, or pulmonic stenosis.
7. Hypertension: systolic blood pressures of 170 mm of mercury or over, or diastolic (fifth phase) pressures of 100 mm of mercury and above, as taken by the physician in the clinic. If the systolic pressure is 180 mm of mercury or over, or the diastolic pressure is 110 mm of mercury or over, as taken by the technician immediately preceding the test, the exercise should not be carried out. If there is a difference of more than 10 mm between the fifth and fourth phase, the fourth phase should be used. If a person states that he is on diuretics for antihypertensive therapy, the exclusion criteria should be lowered by 10 mm of mercury for systolic and diastolic pressure. Persons known to be receiving ganglionic or sympathetic blocking agents are excluded.
8. Insulin therapy.

[2]Appreciation is expressed for the help of Benjamin C. Johnson, M. D., Leon D. Ostrander, M. D., and Park W. Willis III, M. D., in establishing these criteria and the criteria for stopping the exercise.

Table 5.2

MALE TREADMILL TEST POPULATION: PARTICIPATION RATES*

Age Group	Eligible for 3rd Clinical Exam N (1)	Participated in 3rd Clinical Exam N (2)	$\frac{(2)}{(1)}100$ %	Not Available for Treadmill Test** N (3)	$\frac{(3)}{(2)}100$ %	Remainder of Participants in 3rd Exam N (4)	$\frac{(4)}{(2)}100$ %	Medically Examined and Eligible for Treadmill Test N (5)	$\frac{(5)}{(4)}100$ %	Refused Treadmill Test N (6)	$\frac{(6)}{(5)}100$ %	Given Treadmill Test N (7)	$\frac{(7)}{(5)}100$ %
10–14	244	198	81.1	15	7.6	183	92.4	179	97.8	25	14.0	154	86.0
15–19	267	189	70.8	2	1.1	187	98.9	177	94.7	25	14.1	152	85.9
20–24	205	113	55.1	14	12.4	99	87.6	92	92.9	24	26.1	68	73.9
25–34	251	199	79.3	27	13.6	172	86.4	145	84.3	29	20.0	116	80.0
35–44	675	585	86.7	37	6.3	548	93.7	368	67.2	56	15.2	312	84.8
45–54	551	459	83.3	11	2.4	448	97.6	244	54.5	45	18.4	199	81.6
55–69	460	353	76.7	4	1.1	349	98.9	83	23.8	18	21.7	65	78.3
Total	2653	2096	79.0	110	5.2	1986	94.8	1288	64.9	222	17.2	1066	82.8

*This table is approximately correct. There are a few subjects whose status is still not determined, but the final tabulations will not differ appreciably from those shown.

**Although these subjects participated in the third examination, they were not considered for treadmill test because they lived too far away, were misclassified, etc.

Table 5.3

FEMALE TREADMILL TEST POPULATION: PARTICIPATION RATES*

Age Group	Eligible for 3rd Clinical Exam N (1)	Participated in 3rd Clinical Exam N (2)	$100\frac{(2)}{(1)}$ %	Not Available for Treadmill Test** N (3)	$100\frac{(3)}{(2)}$ %	Remainder of Participants in 3rd Exam N (4)	$100\frac{(4)}{(2)}$ %	Examined and Medically Eligible for Treadmill Test N (5)	$100\frac{(5)}{(4)}$ %	Refused Treadmill Test N (6)	$100\frac{(6)}{(5)}$ %	Given Treadmill Test N (7)	$100\frac{(7)}{(5)}$ %
10–14	63	50	79.4	6	12.0	44	88.0	44	100.0	8	18.2	36	81.8
15–19	49	29	59.2	2	6.9	27	93.1	25	92.6	15	60.0	10	40.0
20–24	41	30	73.2	3	10.0	27	90.0	22	81.5	10	45.5	12	54.5
25–34	58	44	75.9	8	18.2	36	81.8	30	83.3	14	46.7	16	53.3
35–44	73	60	82.2	4	6.7	56	93.3	42	75.0	22	52.4	20	47.6
45–54	61	42	68.9	1	2.4	41	97.6	26	63.4	9	34.6	17	65.4
55–69	62	36	58.1	1	2.8	35	97.2	13	37.1	5	38.5	8	61.5
Total	407	291	71.5	25	8.6	266	91.4	202	75.9	83	41.1	119	58.9

*This table is approximately correct. There are a few subjects whose status is still not determined, but the final tabulations will not differ appreciably from those shown.

**Although these subjects participated in the third examination, they were not considered for treadmill test because they lived too far away, were misclassified, etc.

9. Cerebrosvascular accidents or ischemic cerebrovascular episodes, probable or suspect.
10. Any diseases or disabilities that seriously impair walking.

Comparison of Population Samples

The respondents in the 10 percent sample of dwelling units can be expected to be a representative sample of residents in the community. The remaining nine samples were confined to subjects who had been tested previously. The latter group might be biased if new residents to the community or those who moved away are different in the measurements being taken from those people previously examined. If there were only a bias in age distribution, this would not be serious because most analyses are done age-specific. As a last resort, analyses could be restricted to the 10 percent representative sample. However, many more cases would be available if all tested subjects could be included in the analyses.

A possible bias in the treadmill data was investigated by comparing the oxygen uptake measurements of male respondents, age 35 to 39, across all ten living unit samples. The first nine 10 percent samples included only the residents who had been studied in one or both of the previous examinations. The mean responses to the treadmill test ($\dot{V}o_2$ max, ventilation, heart rate, etc.) for males age 35 to 39 in the first nine samples were not different than the average responses for males in the same age group of sample 10.

Next, the exercise responses were studied in the special groups; i.e., males age 10 to 34 who were relatives of coronary heart disease or diabetic cases and relatives of controls.[3] These special groups were not significantly different in metabolic response to the treadmill test from the responses of the age-matched subjects of sample 10.

As a result of these comparisons, it was possible to consider the subjects tested on the treadmill as representative of healthy subjects in the community in the corresponding age groups.

[3]See Chapter 1 for a description of the special groups in the third series of examinations.

Chapter 6 / Response to Treadmill Exercise: Electrocardiographic Changes in Males

Introduction

In 1928, changes in the normal exercise electrocardiogram were observed during an exercised-induced attack of angina pectoris (characteristic severe constricting pain in the chest, possibly radiating to the left arm) (333, p. 296). This shortly led to use of the exercise electrocardiogram in diagnosing coronary heart disease. A very large literature on the exercise electrocardiogram has resulted. An excellent reference is the recent work edited by Blackburn (27). It has long been hypothesized that changes in the ST segment and T-waves during exercise (see Figure 6.1) indicate myocardial ischemia (inadequate circulation to the heart muscle) probably as a result of atherosclerosis of the coronary arteries. This hypothesis has been supported by the observation that breathing gas mixtures with reduced oxygen tensions (10 percent) produces ST segment changes (333, p. 298). Furthermore, recent studies using angiography (X-ray viewing of the coronary arteries) indicate that ST segment (and perhaps ventricular premature beats[1]) are indeed correlated with the presence of atherosclerosis in the coronary arteries (84, 98, 144, 179). Additionally, persons showing ECG changes with exercise are much more likely to develop coronary heart disease than those whose exercise ECG is negative, i.e., normal (84). It is not surprising, therefore, that Simonson (333, p. 295) has concluded that "the electrocardiographic

[1]Arrhythmia reflecting heart irritability.

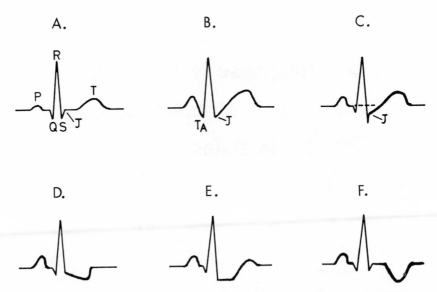

Fig. 6.1 Types of ST-T changes. A : normal ECG, at rest. B : false junctional ST depression resulting from atrial T-wave Ta. C : true junctional ST depression. D : ischemic ST depression, sloping down. E : ischemic ST depression—horizontal. F : isolated T-wave inversion. Reproduced from E. Simonson, "Electrocardiographic stress tolerance tests," in *Progress in Cardiovascular Diseases,* 13 (1970), 269–92, with permission of the author and publisher.

exercise test is the most powerful diagnostic tool available for early detection of coronary artery disease. . . ." What is of particular interest to physical educators is the possibility that physical conditioning reduces the likelihood of observing ECG changes during exercise or raises the threshold when such changes might occur (29, 84, 147, 289).

Electrocardiograms were recorded during exercise in the Tecumseh subject for two reasons. In the first place, observing the electrocardiogram during exercise is an important safety precaution. The exercise was terminated when significant ECG changes occurred. Second, it will be possible in the future to study further the usefulness of the ECG response as an early detector of coronary heart disease.

Results

Relatively few symptoms of any serious degree occurred in the entire study group. None of the persons experienced chest pain after exercise, even if there was ischemic ST segment depression. No instance of severe postexercise hypotension occurred. Fatigue and shortness of breath were the main complaints, and the subjects rarely developed nausea and vomiting after exercise. One person developed persistent vertigo lasting several minutes after the test was completed. Symptoms of moderate to severe leg cramps occurred in twelve persons.

Ischemic ST Segment Depression

All of the subjects who were tested on the treadmill had normal resting electrocardiograms. Nevertheless, 38 of the 1,064, or 3.6 percent, showed horizontal or sagging ST segment depression equal to or greater than 1 mm during and/or after exercise (Figure 6.1D and 6.1E and Table 6.1). This change did not occur in the 427 persons under the age of 29. The

Table 6.1

ST SEGMENT CHANGES

Age (yr)	Total No.	Ischemic ST Depression ≥ 1 mm		Borderline ST Depression 0.5–0.9 mm		J-Junction Depression ≥ 2 mm	
		No.	%	No.	%	No.	%
10–19	304	0	0	0	0	5	1.6
20–29	123	0	0	0	0	7	5.7
30–39	213	6	2.8	2	0.9	18	8.5
40–49	287	17	5.9	7	2.4	17	5.9
50–59	107	10	9.3	2	1.9	10	9.3
60–69	30	5	16.7	2	6.6	4	13.3

Reproduced from (61), *Amer. J. Epidemiol.*, 91 (1970), 372, with permission of the publisher.

frequency of ST segment depression increased progressively from 2.8 percent in the age group 30 to 39 to 16.7 percent in the 60 to 69 group. The majority of the ischemic ST segment depressions were transient and returned to normal soon after exercise. Of the 38 persons who showed ST segment depression, 18 showed this change during and immediately after exercise, 30 showed this change up to 3 minutes after exercise, and only two showed persistent ST segment depression throughout the entire 10-minute recovery period (Table 6.2). Thirty-four of 39 had a negative ST amplitude between 1.0–1.9 mm; only 4 had ST depression greater than 2.0 mm (Table 6.2). Borderline ST segment depression was observed in 13 cases with segmental depression between 0.5–0.9 mm. The frequency of borderline ST segment depression also increased with age (Table 6.1).

J-Junction Depression

J-junction depression equal to or greater than 2 mm with upward slope of ST segment occurred in 61 persons (Figure 6.1C). The frequency

Table 6.2

DURATION AND MAGNITUDE OF ISCHEMIC ST SEGMENT DEPRESSION (*N* = 38)

Duration of ST depression	
ST depression during exercise and immediately after exercise only	18
ST depression return to normal within 3 minutes after exercise	30
Persistent ST depression throughout 10 minute recovery period	2
Delayed ST depression (3 minutes after exercise)	2
Magnitude of ST depression	
−1.0 to −1.5 mm	18
−1.6 to −1.9 mm	16
−2.0 mm or greater	4

Reproduced from (61), *Amer. J. Epidemiol.*, 91 (1970), 372, with permission of the publisher.

also increased with age, from 1.6 percent in the 10 to 19 age group to 13.3 percent in the 60 to 69 age group (Table 6.1).

Ventricular Premature Contractions (VPC) During Exercise

In 69 persons, VPCs occurred during exercise but were absent at rest. Only one person showed a succession of three or more VPCs and another one showed multifocal VPCs. The frequency of VPC during exercise also increased with age, from 1.9 percent in the 20 to 29 age group to 30 percent in the oldest group (Table 6.3). Eight persons showed both VPCs and ischemic ST segment depression.

Table 6.3

VENTRICULAR PREMATURE BEATS DURING EXERCISE

Age (yr)	*Total No.*	*No.*	%
10–19	304	0	0
20–29	213	4	1.9
30–39	123	12	9.8
40–49	287	25	8.7
50–59	107	19	17.8
60–69	30	9	30.0
Total	1,064	69	6.5

Reproduced from (61), *Amer. J. Epidemiol.*, 91 (1970), 373, with permission of the publisher.

Orthostatic T-Wave Changes

Orthostatic T-wave inversions or diphasic T-waves were observed in 49 persons. This is defined as an upright T-wave at sitting position which becomes inverted or diphasic upon standing just before exercise. Such orthostatic T-wave change is a common finding in young persons, but rarely in older persons (Table 6.4). The inverted or diphasic T-wave usually became upright again as exercise went on.

Post-Exercise Giant T-Waves

A post-exercise giant T-wave is defined as a tall, peaked T-wave with an increase of amplitude after exercise of at least 100 percent from the resting T-wave amplitude. The T-waves in such cases have a gradual increase in amplitude during exercise and reach a peak usually one or two minutes after maximal exercise. They gradually return to the original amplitude during the post-exercise recovery period. This is a common finding in young persons. None of the persons over age 50 showed this finding (Table 6.4).

Table 6.4

T-WAVE CHANGES

Age (yr)	Total No.	Orthostatic T-Inversion No.	%	Post-Exercise Giant T No.	%	Post-Exercise T-Inversion No.	%
10–19	304	18	5.9	69	22.7	1	0.3
20–29	123	12	9.6	11	8.9	2	1.6
30–39	213	11	5.2	3	1.4	2	0.9
40–49	287	8	2.8	0	0	6	2.1
50–59	107	0	0	0	0	2	1.8
60–69	30	0	0	0	0	1	3.3
Total	1,064	49	4.6	83	7.8	14	1.3

Reproduced from (61), *Amer. J. Epidemiol.*, 91 (1970), 373, with permission of the publisher.

Post-Exercise T-Inversions

Post-exercise T-wave inversions (Figure 6.1F) occurred in thirteen cases. The frequency of this change is evenly distributed among the various age groups (Table 6.4).

Discussion

Ellestad and co-workers reported that in 284 healthy executives with maximal treadmill exercise, 11 percent developed ischemic ST changes, but chest pain was not associated with this change; while in a group of 236 cardiac patients, 37 percent with positive test had chest pain (113). Bellet and co-workers studied 135 healthy men age 17 to 64 with strenuous exercise;

24.8 percent showed abnormal ECG responses, but none had precordial pain (18). In studies of 268 coronary patients and 346 healthy persons with maximal exercise, 36.2 percent of the patients had chest pain, but only 3.8 percent of healthy persons had chest pain when the exercise was stopped (49). Lloyd-Thomas found that when exercise was continued in physically active anginal patients until the onset of symptoms, chest pain occurred in 139, and ST segment depression was observed in 155 of 187 cases (221).

Post-exertional hypotension has been reported in many studies (22, 59), but none occurred in our group when blood pressure was taken every minute in the 10-minute recovery period. Our subjects were seated immediately after the exercise on a chair placed on the treadmill.

Electrocardiographic changes in healthy men after maximal or near maximal exercise have been reported in many studies. Depending on the age group, method, and intensity of exercise, and criteria for ECG interpretation, the prevalence of ischemic ST segment depression varies from 1 to 10 percent (214). Our data support an age trend of increasing frequency of segment depression in healthy men (4, 18, 22, 84, 85, 199, 319, 346).

The ECG response of ST segment depression after exercise is generally attributed to transient post-exertional myocardial ischemia. It likely reflects functional inadequacy of oxygen transport by coronary circulation, regardless of etiology or structural changes. However, coronary atherosclerosis may account for the majority of cases with post-exercise ST segment depression in persons without other organic lesions of the heart. Mattingly (228) reported on the 10-year follow-up of 980 cases tested by double Master two-step test. A sevenfold increase in the cumulative incidence of myocardial infarction was found in those persons who showed at least 0.5 mm horizontal or down-sloping ST segment depression. Pathologic data obtained at autopsy confirmed the presence of significant coronary atherosclerosis in those with positive ST response after exercise. They found that the sensitivity of the true positive was 84 percent. Only 14 percent showed false negative response and there was no false positive response in persons without coronary atherosclerosis on arteriography (227).

In the present study, although a prevalence of ST segment depression of 3.6 percent was observed, the pattern and magnitude of ST segment depression differs from studies in patients with angina pectoris and/or myocardial infarction. The changes in our study are characterized by their transient nature, usually returning to normal soon after rest and exhibiting less degree in the magnitude of ST segment depression (Table 6.2). A summary of the characteristics of ischemic ST responses in healthy men as compared to coronary patients is shown in Table 6.5.

The significance of occurrence of ventricular premature contractions in isolated form during exercise is uncertain. It is not uncommon in many reported series (18, 31, 214, 346). In a previous study in Tecumseh, it has

Table 6.5

CHARACTERISTICS OF ISCHEMIC ST RESPONSE
IN HEALTHY MEN AS COMPARED
TO CLINICAL CORONARY PATIENTS

	Healthy Men	*Coronary Patients*
Work capacity	Higher	Lower
Chest pain	Usually absent	37%–75%
Ventricular premature beats during exercise	Common	Common
Ischemic ST depression		
Percent	1–10%	> 68%
Magnitude	Shallower	Deeper
Duration	Usually transient	Often persistent

Reproduced from (61), *Amer. J. Epidemiol.*, 91 (1970), 376, with permission of the publisher.

been shown that the prevalence of VPCs at resting ECG also increases with age (62). There was significantly higher prevalence of coronary heart disease in persons with ventricular premature beats than those without, in each age- and sex-specific group (62). Eight of the 38 (21 percent) persons with positive ST responses in the present study showed coexistent ventricular premature beats during exercise.

Post-exercise giant T-waves are common among younger persons (Table 6.4). Usually the maximum was reached one to two minutes after the end of exercise, and gradually returned to original amplitude during the 10-minute recovery period. Simonson has observed such giant T-wave changes in a young person after strenous exercise (331). The significance of this change is unknown. Slight increase in T-wave amplitude has also been observed in cardiac patients, but usually not of such marked degree (331). The changes observed in this study are primarily related to age and intensity of exercise, and apparently not related to cardiac illness or positive ST response. In fact, none of these young persons with post-exercise giant T-waves showed positive ST segment depression. Orthostatic T-wave inversion occurred after the person changed his posture from sitting to standing just before exercise. It usually became upright again as exercise went on. This change is common among young persons. Forty-nine persons in this study showed such changes, and the prevalence decreases with age (Table 6.4). It is not related to positive ST segment response or work capacity. Kemp and Ellestad studied a group of 305 persons with orthostatic and hyperventilative T-wave changes. They found that these changes are common in younger age groups and are not related to ischemic heart disease as evaluated by treadmill exercise test (200).

Chapter *7* / **Response to Treadmill Exercise: Proteinuria**

Introduction

The presence of protein in the urine following strenuous exercise was observed almost a century ago (265) and is now a well-recognized phenomenon (39). The distribution and nature of post-exercise urinary proteins have been described by several investigators (272, 287). Others have studied the relationship between proteinuria and renal function during exercise. However, the relationship between proteinuria and the physiological correlates of stress during exercise—particularly oxygen uptake, maximum heart rate, and systolic blood pressure (at rest and with exercise)—has not been studied in subjects over a wide age range (age 10 to 69) living in a natural community.

Methods

Only 499 of the total 695 males who took the exercise test between November 1967 and January 1969 were included in the present study. This group consisted of only those age 10 to 69 who had a negative pretest proteinuria (285).

The albustix "dip and read" technique was used to measure proteinuria in exercise subjects. Albustix are paper strips impregnated with an indicator dye (tetra bromphenol-blue) which binds protein and causes color changes proportionate to protein concentration in solution. Urinary protein concentration was measured on fresh pre- and post-exercise specimens by albustix strips according to the manufacturer's instructions. Negative and trace concentrations were regarded as negative; all samples showing 1 + or greater were called positive.

It would have been preferable to use biochemical techniques to study proteinuria. However, the field conditions under which this study was performed precluded all but the albustix method. Also, several investigations have shown excellent correlation between this method on the one hand and the sulfsalicylic acid and immunoassay techniques for protein detection on the other (307).

Results

The decade-specific incidence of proteinuria after exercise increased with age (Table 7.1) until the fourth decade. The explanation for the lower incidence of proteinuria in men age 40 to 49 is that they were not maximally exercised, unlike younger individuals. There are too few individuals in the group over age 49 with proteinuria for satisfactory analysis.

In Table 7.2 the means for (1) weight (kg), (2) oxygen consumption (with heart rate of 150 bpm), (3) maximum heart rate, (4) systolic blood pressure at rest, (5) systolic blood pressure during exercise (at heart rate of 150 bpm), (6) total exercise time, and (7) oxygen consumption ml/kg of body weight (at heart rate of 150 bpm) are compared for the groups with and without post-exercise proteinuria. The trend is toward higher mean values for each of the parameters in the proteinuric individuals.

Covariance analysis (holding age constant) shows that oxygen consump-

Table 7.1

AGE INCIDENCE OF PROTEINURIA DURING EXERCISE

Decade	Total Tested	No Urine Sample Available	Positive Pre-Exercise Proteinuria (Excluded)	Total in Study (Negative Pre-Exercise Proteinuria)	Total with Post-Exercise Proteinuria	Percent with Proteinuria Post-Exercise
10–19	206	36	18	152	11	7.2
20–29	79	11	1	67	9	13.2
30–39	139	19	3	117	23	19.6
40–49	191	24	4	163	10	6.5
50–59	62	12	1	49	1	2.4
60–69	18	1	1	16	0	0
Total	695	103	28	499	53	10.6

Reproduced from (285) with permission of the publisher.

Table 7.2

COMPARISON OF INDIVIDUALS WITH AND WITHOUT PROTEINURIA DURING EXERCISE WITH RESPECT TO SEVERAL PHYSIOLOGICAL VARIABLES

Age by Decade	Variable	Proteinuria Absent			Proteinuria Present		
		Mean	*SD*	*N*	*Mean*	*SD*	*N*
10–19	Weight (kg)	57.9	17.5	141	71.5	8.8	11
	$\dot{V}O_2$ (Liters)—HR = 150 bpm	1.75	0.52	141	2.26	0.32	11
	Max. HR	186.6	13.6	141	192.5	9.7	11
	SBP—Rest	122.9	11.2	141	128.2	12.3	11
	SBP HR = 150 bpm	168.0	22.1	135	175.3	19.6	11
	Total Time Exercise	22.70		135	26.16		11
	$\dot{V}O_2$ (ml/kg)—HR = 150 bpm	31.04	7.25	141	31.76	3.37	11
20–29	Weight (kg)	76.6	11.9	58	85.8	9.2	9
	$\dot{V}O_2$ (Liters)—HR = 150 bpm	2.19	0.37	57	2.48	0.21	9
	Max. HR	186.1	14.2	57	178.2	15.3	9
	SBP—Rest	130.8	13.1	58	138.9	13.8	9
	SBP HR = 150 bpm	187.0	16.8	58	204.0	19.4	9
	Total Time Exercise	22.43		57	21.38		9
	$\dot{V}O_2$ (ml/kg)—HR = 150 bpm	28.88	3.68	57	29.00	2.31	9
30–39	Weight (kg)	76.9	10.2	94	81.2	10.4	23
	$\dot{V}O_2$ (Liters)—HR = 150 bpm	2.09	0.35	94	2.31	0.34	23
	Max. HR	176.6	15.7	93	183.3	12.1	23
	SBP—Rest	130.8	12.1	94	133.4	11.0	23
	SBP HR = 150 bpm	190.6	17.3	91	199.0	16.5	23
	Total Time Exercise	19.35		91	21.29		23
	$\dot{V}O_2$ (ml/kg)—HR = 150 bpm	22.43	4.17	94	28.67	3.93	23
40–49	Weight (kg)	78.8	12.2	153	83.3	13.7	10
	$\dot{V}O_2$ (Liters)—HR = 150 bpm	2.18	0.40	150	2.30	0.34	10
	Max. HR	155.5	11.7	153	160.4	7.5	10
	SBP—Rest	133.6	14.3	151	128.2	10.2	10
	SBP HR = 150 bpm	200.1	21.2	143	201.4	19.1	10
	Total Time Exercise	15.34		141	15.68		10
	$\dot{V}O_2$ (ml/kg)—HR = 150 bpm	27.94	4.80	150	27.95	3.89	10

Abbreviations used in table:
$\dot{V}O_2$—*oxygen uptake*
Max. HR—maximum heart rate
SBP—systolic blood pressure
$\dot{V}O_2$ *(ml/kg)—HR = 150 bpm—oxygen consumption (ml/kg) at heart rate of 150 beats per minute.*
Reproduced from (285) with permission of the publisher.

tion (at standard heart rate of 150 bpm), maximum heart rate, systolic blood pressure (at heart rate of 150 bpm), and total time of exercise were significantly correlated ($p < .01$) with the occurrence of post-exercise proteinuria (Table 7.3). Weight was also significantly correlated with the phenomenon but at a lower level of significance ($p < .05$). There was no statistically significant correlation with systolic blood pressure at rest or with oxygen uptake per kg (at heart rate of 150 bpm).

All of the factors found to be correlated in this study with the occurrence

Table 7.3

COVARIANCE ANALYSIS (HOLDING AGE CONSTANT) OF SEVERAL
FACTORS AND THEIR RELATIONSHIP TO THE
OCCURRENCE OF EXERCISE PROTEINURIA

Factor	F	sig.
$\dot{V}O_2$ (Liters)—HR = 150 bpm	25.8	$p < .01$
Total Time of Exercise	11.6	$p < .01$
Maximum Heart Rate Reached (bpm)	9.1	$p < .01$
Systolic Blood Pressure	8.7	$p < .01$
Weight	3.6	$p < .05$
Systolic Blood Pressure (at rest)	1.8	$p > .05$
$\dot{V}O_2$ (ml/kg)—HR = 150 bpm	.3	$p > .05$

Reproduced from (285) with permission of the publisher.

of proteinuria can be related to the physiological stress imposed by exercise on an individual. This supports other investigations that exercise intensity and proteinuria are related (155, 186, 207). These factors (in decreasing order of *F* value by covariate analysis) are oxygen uptake at heart rate of 150 bpm, total time of exercise, maximum heart rate reached, systolic blood pressure (at heart rate of 150 bpm), and weight. Some of these factors are related inversely to physical fitness.

The mechanism by which protein appears in the urine as a result of exercise is not completely clear. Castenfors (54) has summarized the physiological factors associated with exercise proteinuria. These include a decreased renal plasma flow during exercise, increase in filtration fraction, decrease in urine flow, increase in glomerular permeability, renal vasoconstriction, and possibly an increase in renin activity by direct sympathetic stimulation.

All of the measurements related to the occurrence of proteinuria probably operate through the mechanism of increasing glomerular load or permeability as discussed above. Increased blood pressure during exercise may force more protein through the glomerulus than can be reabsorbed. Such pressure increases may also alter the shape of glomerular pores, with more protein leaking into the glomerular filtrate. Other factors (such as heart rate, oxygen uptake, and time of exercise) may simply be related to increased blood pressure, or they may increase glomerular permeability by effects on body temperature, hormonal secretion, or acid-base balance as for example by the activation of kallikrein (265). The precise mechanisms of these changes require further investigation.

8 / Response to Treadmill Exercise: Age and Attainment of a "Steady State"

Introduction

In many work capacity tests, a "steady state" is assumed, and in most methods of measuring cardiac output during exercise this condition is a requirement for precise results. Nevertheless, there is still confusion as to what constitutes a steady state and how much time is required to attain it. Few data have been published on the minute-by-minute physiological adjustments at various exercise intensities, and age differences in these adjustments have rarely been reported.

Method

The treadmill test and the physiological parameters which were monitored were described in Chapter 5. For purposes of the present analysis, 50 of the 1,064 male subjects were selected at random from various age groups (153, 252). The age distribution and body weights are summarized in Table 8.1. Data were recorded throughout the treadmill test on all subjects. However, usually the measurements were made on the recordings only during the last minute of each treadmill grade. For purposes of the present report—that is, for studying adjustment at each level, the measurements were made over the last 30 seconds of each of the 3 minutes at each grade. The six physiological measures being reported include: oxygen uptake, heart rate, carbon

Table 8.1

DESCRIPTIVE STATISTICS OF SUBJECTS

Age Group	Number of Subjects	Age (Years)		Weight (Kilograms)	
		Mean	Range	Mean	Range
10–19	10	14.2	11–18	56.1	38–81
20–39	20	29.1	20–38	76.6	57–95
40–59	15	47.5	40–56	78.0	59–106
60–65	5	62.2	60–65	74.6	65–83

Reproduced from (153) with permission of the publisher.

dioxide production, ventilation, oxygen pulse, and respiratory exchange ratio (i.e., ratio of carbon dioxide produced to oxygen consumed).

Because it was thought the naiveté of the subjects with regard to exercise tests might have an effect on the results, the author (HJM, age 48 at the time), who has taken treadmill exercise tests on many occasions, took this particular test four times during a period of several months. The data for him are also discussed. He exercised to a grade of 27 percent on two occasions and 24 percent on the other trials. The times in minutes were 26.0, 27.8, 28.3, and 28.2. The maximal oxygen uptakes in ml/kg/min were 48, 47, 47, and 49.

Results

The mean values for the various physiological measurements during the last 30 seconds of each minute of the various exercise levels for the four age groups are plotted in Figures 8.1 to 8.3. The terminal points on these graphs do not represent the duration of exercise of all subjects. A few of the more fit subjects exercised a little longer than the average so the number of subjects used to calculate the means in these graphs decreased in a few instances as the test continued. The number of cases in each instance is shown in Table 8.2. The subjects 60 years of age and older walked longer, on the average, than the 40 to 59 year age group. This occurred because, as noted above, the treadmill speed was reduced to 2 mph for these older subjects.

In Table 8.2 it will be noted that the number of subjects participating in each age group varied slightly from level to level. This variation was because of loss of data during the test. All subjects worked continuously on the treadmill; however, at times it was found necessary to remove the mouthpiece for a short period of time to communicate with the subject. This meant that ventilation and gas concentrations could not be measured during this period. The period lasted no more than 30 seconds, but, because in this analysis the major consideration was the number of adjustments during work at a given level, all data for this subject during that level were excluded. Each level, therefore, had the same subjects performing for those three minutes. With subject HJM, the mouthpiece was not removed during the test.

Oxygen Uptake

Figure 8.1 shows that by the second minute at each grade, oxygen uptake plateaued. In some instances, particularly at the lower grades, there

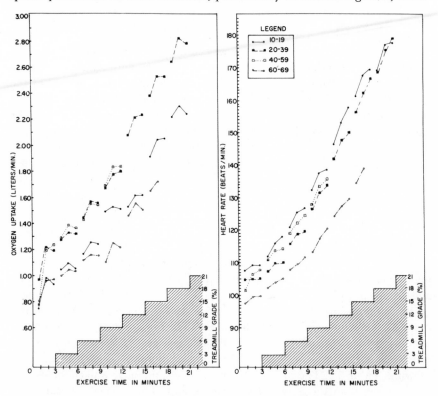

Fig. 8.1 Oxygen uptake (left side) and heart rate (right side). Each point represents the mean for the particular age group. Reproduced from (153) with permission of the publisher.

was a tendency to "overshoot" so that oxygen uptake decreased in the third minute. The pattern was the same in all four age groups and in the experienced subject (HJM). An overshoot in some instances is not unexpected because a change of 3 percent in treadmill grade necessitates a considerable change in the mechanics of walking and it is conceivable that more than a

Table 8.2   NUMBER OF SUBJECTS USED TO CALCULATE MEANS IN FIGURES 8.1 TO 8.3

Physiological Parameter	Age Groups	Minutes of Exercise																				
		1	2	3	4	5	6	7	8	9	10	11	12	13	14	15	16	17	18	19	20	21
Heart Rate	10–19	10	10	10	10	10	10	9	9	9	10	10	10	9	9	9	9	9	9	7	7	7
	20–39	19	19	19	20	20	20	20	20	20	20	20	20	20	20	20	19	19	19	14	14	14
	40–59	14	14	14	15	15	15	15	15	15	14	14	14									
	60–65	5	5	5	5	5	5	5	5	5	5	5	5									
Ventilation	10–19	9	9	9	10	10	10	10	10	10	9	9	9	8	8	8	8	8	8	5	5	5
Resp. Freq.	20–39	18	18	18	19	19	19	20	20	20	17	17	17	16	16	16	14	14	14	12	12	12
Resp. Exchange Ratio	40–59	13	13	13	14	14	14	13	13	13	12	12	12									
Oxygen Uptake	60–65	4	4	4	5	5	5	5	5	5	4	4	4	3	3	3	5	5				
Oxygen Pulse	10–19	9	9	9	10	10	10	10	10	10	9	9	9	7	7	7	7	8	8	8	6	6
	20–39	18	18	18	19	19	19	20	20	20	17	17	17	16	16	16	14	14	14	12	12	12
	40–59	13	13	13	14	14	14	13	13	13	12	12	12									
	60–65	4	4	4	5	5	5	5	5	5	4	4	4	3	3	3		5				

Reproduced from (153) with permission of the publisher.

69

minute or two might be needed to make the adjustments. Even at the highest workloads, the oxygen uptake generally reached a peak by the second minute.

Heart Rate

Figure 8.1 indicates that heart rate did not reach a steady state except in the younger subjects and then only at the very lowest workloads. In the experienced subject, during the first two workloads, the heart rate was approximately in a steady state. However, at each of the other loads, heart rate increased throughout the three minutes, similar to what was seen in Figure 8.1.

Oxygen Pulse

Figure 8.2 shows that oxygen pulse increases with an increase in strenuousness (grade level) of the exercise. At a given workload, because oxygen uptake during the second and third minute is essentially constant

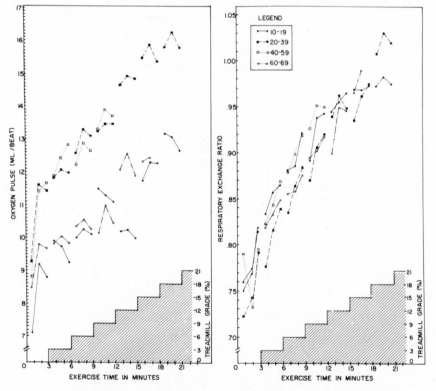

Fig. 8.2 Oxygen pulse (left side) and respiratory exchange ratio (right side). Each point represents the mean for the particular age group. Reproduced from (153) with permission of the publisher.

and heart rate continued to increase, oxygen pulse decreased slightly in all age groups and also in the experienced subject.

Carbon Dioxide Production

Carbon dioxide production is shown in Figure 8.3. There is a tendency for CO_2 production to approach a plateau at each load, but this is not nearly as pronounced as in the case of oxygen uptake. The result is an increase in respiratory exchange ratio during the three minutes at most workloads (Figure 8.2). Age of subject is not related to this phenomenon.

Ventilation

There was a tendency for ventilation to approach a steady state at low workloads, but at higher grades there was no evidence of this (Figure 8.3). There were no clear age differences and the experienced subject showed the same pattern. Respiratory frequency (not shown) was less consistent but at lower workloads the rate leveled off or decreased in the third minute. At

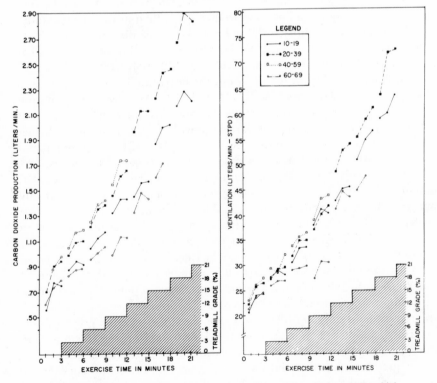

Fig. 8.3 Carbon dioxide production (left side) and ventilation (right side). Each point represents the mean for the particular age group. Reproduced from (153) with permission of the publisher.

higher loads, no steady state was approached. There were no consistent differences in age groups.

Discussion

Most investigators have reported that a steady state in oxygen uptake is reached in fixed-load exercise within a few minutes over a wide range of strenuousness of work (56, 94, 126, 143, 168, 217, 266). This is essentially what we observed. However, some reports showed a rapid adjustment at low workloads and slower adjustment at high workloads (102, 363, 371), and in one investigation (12) using five subjects, the opposite was true; more rapid adjustment at higher workloads. In one study of constant speed, strenuous running to exhaustion within 3 minutes, the oxygen consumption decreased in the second minute and then increased markedly in the last 30 seconds as exhaustion was approached (316). This was more strenuous exercise with less time for adjustment to take place than in the present study.

Heart rate in our subjects did not reach a plateau by the third minute at almost all workloads. Except for one report (16), this agrees with what others have observed (12, 25, 42, 126, 155, 170, 184, 229, 329, 363). In prolonged fixed-load work (60 minutes), the heart rate has been reported to be still rising at end of work (68, 77, 111, 112, 151). Although cardiac output was not measured in the present study, previous investigations indicate that at low levels of work a steady state is reached within $1^1/_2$ minutes and at higher workloads within about 3 minutes (56, 126, 143, 183, 184) except in patients in whom cardiac output increases more slowly in response to exercise (25, 170, 183, 184). However, in some normal subjects a steady state in cardiac output was not achieved in 3 to 4 minutes. In prolonged work, cardiac output remained fairly constant but because heart rate increased, stroke volume decreased (111, 112). Our decrease in oxygen pulse during the third minute of a particular workload can be similarly explained. Although a change in arteriovenous oxygen difference can not be ruled out as a factor, the decrease in O_2 uptake and increase in heart rate could account for the change in O_2 pulse during the third minute. The increase in oxygen pulse with an increase in treadmill grade, which we observed, is likely due *primarily* to an increase in arteriovenous oxygen difference as the workload becomes greater (142).

Harris and Porter (155) measured heart rate and esophageal temperature during 10-minute periods of work at various treadmill grades. Only at the lowest grades (mild work) did the temperature and heart rate not increase. They attributed the gradually increasing heart rates at the other workloads to an increase in body temperature and in the early minutes of more strenuous work to an additional factor, the accumulation of lactic acid in the blood.

The results of Shephard (329) and Saiki and colleagues (321) suggest that the continued rise in heart rate beyond the first few minutes is not due to lactic acid production. In prolonged submaximal work, body temperature increases throughout the hour of exercise in a controlled and comfortable environment (111, 112, 148, 315). It is possible that an increase in body temperature might contribute to the increase in heart rate during the 3 minutes at a given treadmill grade. The interesting experiments by Webb and Luft (364) and by Jose and others (185) raise doubts that this is the case. In the first of these studies the core temperature was prevented from rising by water cooling and still the heart rate increased. In the second investigation (185) the intrinsic heart rate was studied by means of injections of propranolol and atropine. Under these conditions, an increase in heart rate during exercise could not be accounted for by an increase in body temperature. As workload increases, a little more oxygen debt is accumulated (8) and this might explain the increase in heart rate in our tests, although, of course, there could be neurogenic and hormonal factors involved.

At low workloads, ventilation in liters per minute is reported to reach a steady state in 3 to 4 minutes (8, 56, 94, 217), but not during more strenuous work (18, 56, 102, 168). This is essentially what was observed in the present study. Carbon dioxide production required more time to reach a plateau than did oxygen uptake in our subjects. Hence, the respiratory exchange ratio increased during this adjustment period. These observations support those of others (8, 56, 277). There appeared to be no age differences in this phenomenon. Norris and co-workers similarly reported no effect of age (277).

The rate of acquisition of a steady state at any given load has been thought to be related to physical fitness of the subjects. Dill and others (102) observed ten subjects who ran for 20 minutes on a treadmill at 9.3 km/hr. The four who had accumulated the most blood lactate (hence, the least fit) required longer to achieve a steady state in various physiological measurements. This agrees with the conclusions of Wasserman and collaborators (363, 371). Brouha (42), in an experiment in which the subject pedalled a bicycle ergometer at constant load for 200 minutes, reported that the heart rate did not level off until the end of the ride when the subject was in an untrained state. After 84 days of training, although the heart rate was lower throughout, it still required about 12 minutes to reach a steady state. Harris and Porter (155) concluded the heart rate would reach a steady state sooner in more fit people only if the fit person is able to lose heat faster during exercise.

In the present study, as the treadmill test continued and the workload increased, some of the subjects could no longer continue; hence the decrease in number of subjects in Table 8.2. In order to determine the effect of this, the various measurements were analyzed for only those subjects who completed the highest workload in each age group. These were obviously the more fit subjects. A comparison of their graphs with Figures 8.1 through

8.3 indicated that, although the responses of heart rate and ventilation at a given workload were lower for the more fit subjects, the physiological adjustment during the 3 minutes at each workload was not different from the group as a whole. It may be that a period of more than 3 minutes is required before an effect of fitness on rate of acquisition of a steady state would be observed. It is also more likely that the effect of fitness of the subject on the time required to achieve a steady state may only be seen when the work is more strenuous, as was the case in the report by Dill and collaborators (102). Indeed, Jones and others (183) presented evidence in young men that the correlation between fitness and rapidity with which a steady state is achieved at high workloads is moderately good $(r = .76)$ but not at low workloads $(r = .23)$.

It appears that the physiological adjustments associated with achieving a "steady state" during exercise, including heart rate, are not clearly understood. Age does not appear to be an important factor in these adjustments.

Chapter 9 / Physical Fitness of School Children

If a muscle is exercised, it hypertrophies and becomes stronger. If a sedentary person undertakes a conditioning program, his work capacity increases. In short, exercise programs improve our ability to do exercise. This has been expressed in another way: nature is neither cruel nor kind, simply obedient.

The question of whether resistance to disease or disability improves with an increase in fitness as a result of exercise is another question. In order to provide some data that bear on this, a battery of fitness tests was administered to most of the school children in the Tecumseh Community Health Study. The primary objectives were (a) to correlate the fitness results with risk factors associated with predisposition to disease, (b) to determine, in a longitudinal study, if children who are more fit have a different susceptibility to disease and disability later in life than those who are less fit. It may also be possible to obtain answers to other questions, as for example, whether the exercise habits and leisure activities in later life are related to physical fitness in school, and whether family environment has an effect on fitness or exercise habits. The longitudinal aspects of the study must await the passage of time. The relationship of physical fitness to laboratory measurements associated with certain diseases will be reported in later sections of this monograph. This chapter will contain analyses of the physical fitness data which may be of interest and value to those planning and conducting school programs.

Physical Fitness Tests

It is virtually impossible to obtain complete consensus of opinion with regard to the definition of physical fitness.[1] A debate of these issues is not appropriate here. Probably the most generally accepted battery of simple tests, certainly the most widely used, is the group of tests used in a national survey endorsed by the American Association for Health, Physical Education and Recreation (AAHPER) (176).

Fitness Tests Administered in 1966

The AAHPER tests have been administered to more than 25 million American children. Included in this battery are pullups (bent arm-hang for girls), standing long jump (i.e., broad jump), a shuttle run, situps, 50-yard dash, softball throw for distance, and a 600-yard run-walk. This entire AAHPER battery of tests was administered to school children in Tecumseh in 1966. In addition, because of the relation thought to exist between low back pain and strength and flexibility in the trunk (208), a trunk flexion (326) and trunk extension test (91) were also given to these children in 1966. All the children, with a few exceptions, were tested. In some instances it was necessary to reschedule some children three or four times because they were so reluctant to be tested that they purposely missed school on those days. Those who were not tested included boys or girls whose medical condition did not permit it and a few who refused and whose parents requested that they not be tested. In addition, for medical reasons, some children were not tested on particular items. In all, 2,060 children (938 girls and 1,122 boys) in Tecumseh were tested by a trained team from the University of Michigan.[2] This represents approximately 99 percent of the children in grades 4 to 12. The directions outlined in the AAHPER Youth Fitness Test Manual (176, 379) were followed exactly except for the softball throw, in which case the distance was measured to the closest yard rather than the closest foot. There is enough variability among subjects for the closest yard to be sufficiently precise. Precautions were taken to insure uniformity of the procedures, instructions, and measurements.

Step Test

In addition to the fitness tests listed above, the modified Harvard Step Test described in Chapter 4 was administered to most of these same

[1]Reference is made here to the practical tests that can be used in the public schools. There is much better understanding and agreement concerning the more sophisticated laboratory tests, such as the treadmill test described earlier.

[2]Appreciation is expressed to G. Canamere, D. A. Cunningham, J. Davis, T. Fagan, N. Hart, J. Harvey, R. Hermiston, G. Howard, B. Kiebler, A. J. Kozar, S. Loebs, B. Montoye, J. Polley, J. Stovall, and G. Wade for help in the testing.

children during the second series of examinations in 1961 to 1965. On the average, the step test was given 26 months (range 9 to 47 months) before the other fitness tests. It was, therefore, necessary to correct the step test scores for age and interval between data-collection periods by analysis of covariance or regression analysis.

Value of Age, Height, and Weight in Establishing Fitness Standards

Classification schemes, mainly based on age, height, and weight, have been in use in the United States since almost the beginning of this century (152). Classification indices of various kinds have been used principally for two purposes: (a) for grouping boys and girls into roughly homogeneous groups for athletic competition or instruction and (b) as a basis for establishing achievement standards in various fitness tests or sports skills. The analysis that follows concerns the use of classification indices for the second purpose. A more detailed analysis has been published elsewhere (250).

It is well-known that fitness tests of various kinds are generally not highly correlated. If they were, one test would suffice. If the various tests measure different qualities, most of the useful information is lost when the fitness of children or adults is expressed by some composite score. The situation would be similar to averaging results of a group of medical tests. Would an individual be in the fiftieth percentile by virtue of having exceptionally fine teeth and exceptionally poor peripheral circulation? Similarly, the average of a poor score in strength with an excellent score in flexibility would provide little useful information for guidance if the individual's two scores are buried in an average score. Fortunately, in recent years this has been recognized; for example, standards for *individual items* in the Youth Fitness Survey are provided (176, 379). This is an important concept with regard to the use of a classification index because it then becomes essential to know the relationships between the elements that enter into a classification scheme, on the one hand, and each individual test item, on the other. Otherwise, some children might be penalized through the use of such an index.

It is a common practice in the schools to use combinations of age, height, weight, and grade to establish standards of performance for physical education activities. In both national surveys of youth fitness in the United States, percentile standards were reported by age and by classification system based on age, height, and weight (176, 379). The superiority of the latter method was implied (379, p. 15). However, because achievement standards based on age and sex alone are simpler to calculate and simpler to interpret and explain to students and parents, we questioned whether the use of body stature and weight in addition to age and sex is of sufficient value to merit the additional time and effort. The fitness test scores obtained in 1966 for the children in Tecumseh were used to obtain an answer to this question.

Ordered stepwise regression was one method employed in the analysis. The results are shown in Table 9.1. The first column of figures indicates the percentage of the variance in the fitness scores associated with age. Thus, the first line indicates that about 24 percent of the variance in pullups in boys is associated with age of the subject. If height is added we are now able to account for 26 percent, and if the multiple regression is based on age, height, and weight, 33 percent of the variance in the pullup scores is accounted for.

The inclusion of weight in a classification index could be questioned regardless of its correlation with the other measurements because part of the weight is constituted by bone and muscle, but part is also attributed to fat. To illustrate, if the effects of height and age are removed, the remaining negative partial correlation coefficients between weight and performance in the runs or pullups (bent arm-hang) in boys and girls are significant.

Table 9.1

SQUARED COEFFICIENTS OF DETERMINATION (DECIMAL OMITTED)
BETWEEN FITNESS SCORES (DEPENDENT VARIABLE) AND
INDEPENDENT VARIABLES: ENTRY-ORDERED (1)
AGE (2) HEIGHT AND (3) WEIGHT

	Dependent Variable With:		
	Age	*Age and Height*	*Age, Height, and Weight*
Boys:			
Pullups	24	26	33
Trunk Flexion	5	5	5
Trunk Extension	14	17	18
Long Jump	52	55	58
Shuttle Run	40	41	45
Situps	6	7	10
50-yd Run	53	55	59
Softball Throw	55	61	61
600-yd Run	43	45	53
Girls:			
Arm-Hang	0	1	18
Trunk Flexion	6	6	7
Trunk Extension	13	16	17
Long Jump	14	18	26
Shuttle Run	13	17	24
Situps	2	2	7
50-yd Run	22	26	36
Softball Throw	26	29	29
600-yd Run	6	7	25

Reproduced from (250) with permission of the publisher.

This is likely due, in part at least, to excess fat in some of the children. By considering body weight in the classification index, one is then, to some extent, giving the advantage to fat children—that is, raising the percentile scores rather than allowing the excess fat to lower the relative performance or score.

A study of Table 9.1 will indicate that in the case of boys, age and height or a combination of age, height, and weight accounts for very little more of the variance than simply age alone. In the case of girls, this is also true for most of the tests with regard to the addition of height. The addition of weight, however, accounts for considerably more of the variance in the flexed arm-hang, the 600-yard run, the standing broad jump, and the 50-yard run than does age and height alone. In almost every case, weight is negatively related to performance when age and height are partialled out. Arm strength and speed over the ground as measured in these tests is thought of in terms of one's ability to move his own body weight. Correcting for body weight (i.e., including weight in a classification index) is therefore a questionable procedure.

In the case of the boys, it is quite clear that if achievement standards are developed for each age, it is not necessary to be concerned about differences in height or weight among the children. With regard to girls, age is less closely related to performance. This is to be expected from the age curves in the original youth fitness survey reports (176, 379). However, even with girls, age accounts for almost as much of the variance in fitness scores as does age and height. In the standing long jump, the shuttle run, and the 50-yard run, height makes its greatest contributions, but even in these instances the increase in the amount of variance accounted for by the addition of height is only 4 percent. To demonstrate this in a very practical way, age-specific percentile ranks were developed for girls in these events. Next the girls within each age group were subdivided into two groups using the median height as the dividing point. Percentile ranks were then developed for the lower half of the height distribution and also for the upper half, for each age group. Results of two representative ages for one event, standing long jump, are shown in Table 9.2. If we disregard height, we would use the middle column marked "all subjects." A girl, age 11, whose standing long jump score is 52 inches would be at the fiftieth percentile. If, on the other hand, she were in the lower half of the class in stature, we would use the left-hand column in age group 11. In this instance, 52 inches in the broad jump would still place her at the fiftieth percentile. If she were among the taller girls in the class, a score of 52 inches would place her in the forty-fifth percentile when compared to other girls in this half of the height distribution. Thus, if we were to develop two percentile achievement standards, one for the taller and one for the shorter girls, it would make a difference of about 5 percentile points. This is also true of the other events and various age groups.

Table 9.2

PERCENTILE RANKS FOR THE STANDING LONG JUMP (IN INCHES)
GIRLS: AGE 11 AND 15

Percentile	Age 11			Age 15		
	Lower Half of Height Distribution	*All Subjects*	*Upper Half of Height Distribution*	*Lower Half of Height Distribution*	*All Subjects*	*Upper Half of Height Distribution*
95	66	67	68	77	78	79
90	64	64	65	73	74	75
85	60	61	63	71	70	69
80	60	60	61	68	68	68
75	59	59	60	65	64	64
70	59	59	59	64	64	63
65	56	58	58	64	63	61
60	54	56	56	63	61	60
55	53	54	55	61	60	60
50	52	52	54	59	59	58
45	50	51	52	58	57	57
40	48	49	50	55	55	55
35	48	48	49	55	55	55
30	45	47	48	53	54	54
25	45	45	46	51	52	53
20	44	44	44	50	51	51
15	43	43	43	49	49	49
10	40	41	41	46	46	43
5	38	38	37	44	41	37
N=	67	132	65	55	107	52

Reproduced from (250) with permission of the publisher.

It appears clear, therefore, that one can disregard height and/or weight if achievement standards are established for specific ages and for boys and girls separately. This is essentially the conclusion of Gross and Casiani (152) and Espenschade (121), who used somewhat different approaches to the problem.

Physical Fitness and Present Enrollment in Physical Education

Credit requirement for physical education in high school varies among the states, depending in part on the laws enacted. There is also considerable variability in the requirement within a state. It is not uncommon for physical education to be an elective for one, two, or even all four years. It was the purpose of the present investigation to compare some aspects of physical fitness of high school children who elect to take physical education with those who do not. Tecumseh has one high school (grades 9 to 12) with an enrollment of 894. The students are required to take one elective (minor) each semester in addition to the "solids" taken. The elective must be chosen from among art, band, chorus, and physical education; and any combination is possible during the four years, including eight semesters in one area.

In a previous study (335) comparison of the fitness of physical education participants and nonparticipants was made among college women. As might be expected, the participants were superior in some aspects of fitness. Thirty years before, a similar comparison among college women was made in which participants were superior in attitudes, knowledge, and general motor ability (326). Apparently this kind of study has not been done in a comprehensive way among high school students.

Fitness Tests, 1966

All the children, with a few exceptions, were tested. Those who were not ($N = 9$) included boys or girls whose medical condition did not permit it and a few who refused and whose parents requested they not be tested. There were nine students over 18 years of age and two under 14 who were tested but whose data were not included in the analysis because of the small numbers in these age groups.

The children were grouped according to whether they were enrolled in physical education, chorus, band, or art at the time the tests were administered. The N in this analysis was slightly less than the total N of 874 because in some instances a student was exempt from the elective plan (transfers, for example). The mean fitness scores for the various groups were compared. To adjust for any differences in age distribution in the four groups, analysis of covariance was employed with age as the covariant. The .05 level was accepted for significance in all analyses. The age-adjusted means are presented in Table 9.3. Except for trunk extension for boys, all of the F-values (analysis of covariance) were significant, indicating that the mean fitness scores for the various groups were significantly different.

A comparison of mean fitness scores of the individual groups is presented in Table 9.4. Duncan's New Multiple Range Test was used to determine which differences were significant. Among the boys, the group electing physical education had the highest mean scores in all tests and in most instances differences were significant. The band group was next and usually their mean scores were significantly lower than the physical education group, but significantly greater than either the chorus or art group. There were no significant differences between the last two groups except in the 600-yard run, in which the chorus group was better than the art group.

The results for girls were only slightly different. The physical education group scored best except in the bent arm-hang and the trunk extension, where the band group was superior, but not significantly so. Except for the two tests just mentioned, the band group scored second highest in all tests. The chorus group ranked third and the art group last in all tests.

Table 9.3

AGE-ADJUSTED MEANS BY SEX AND HIGH SCHOOL ELECTIVES

Test	Boys				Girls			
	PE (N = 234)	*Chorus (N = 14)*	*Band (N = 86)*	*Art (N = 26)*	*PE (N = 167)*	*Chorus (N = 35)*	*Band (N = 43)*	*Art (N = 40)*
Pullups (number)	5.02	2.13	3.25	2.04				
Arm-Hang (seconds)					8.25	6.66	8.79	6.33
Flexion (inches)	10.38	9.29	10.32	10.20	12.31	11.39	11.98	10.05
Extension (inches)	16.90	16.34	16.73	16.59	18.01	16.99	18.21	16.64
Long Jump (inches)	77.07	67.39	72.11	65.78	62.10	55.52	56.13	53.80
Shuttle Run (seconds)	9.86	11.15	10.31	10.70	11.07	11.73	11.62	11.87
Situps (number)	84.87	44.02	57.31	45.05	30.79	23.73	27.09	19.90
50-Yd Dash (seconds)	7.07	7.76	7.34	7.88	8.16	8.49	8.40	8.60
Softball Throw (feet)	162.2	125.4	161.8	136.1	82.4	71.59	76.68	67.32
600-Yd Run (seconds)	112.6	132.4	120.2	138.5	157.8	184.4	168.9	194.4

Table 9.4

DUNCAN'S NEW MULTIPLE RANGE TEST:
COMPARISON OF MEAN FITNESS SCORES

Test	Electives[a]							
	Boys				Girls			
Pullups (bent arm-hang)	PE	Band	Chorus	Art	Band	PE	Chorus	Art
Trunk Flexion	PE	Band	Art	Chorus	PE	Band	Chorus	Art
Trunk Extension	PE	Band	Art	Chorus	Band	PE	Chorus	Art
Long Jump	PE	Band	Chorus	Art	PE	Band	Chorus	Art
Shuttle Run	PE	Band	Art	Chorus	PE	Band	Chorus	Art
Situps	PE	Band	Art	Chorus	PE	Band	Chorus	Art
50-Yd Dash	PE	Band	Chorus	Art	PE	Band	Chorus	Art
Softball Throw	PE	Band	Art	Chorus	PE	Band	Chorus	Art
600-Yd Run	PE	Band	Chorus	Art	PE	Band	Chorus	Art

[a]*The group with the best age-adjusted mean score is on left, the group with the second best score is in the next column, and so on. If two or more groups are not joined by a line below, the difference(s) is/are significant ($p < .05$).*

Step Test Results

The results of the comparison in exercise heart rate (at 2.5 minutes of a 3-minute submaximal test) are shown in the left side of Figure 9.1. All of these means are adjusted for age and period between data collection. In both boys and girls, the heart rates were lower (more fit) among the physical education and band groups. Analysis of covariance and the Duncan's New Multiple Range Test indicated the differences between the means of

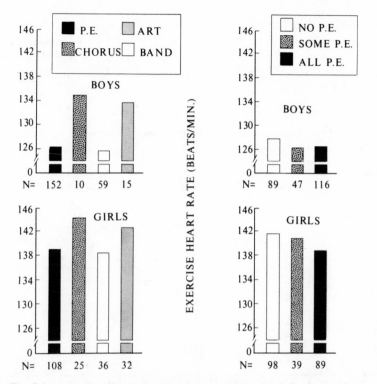

Fig. 9.1 Left side: The relationship of current high school elective and heart rate response to a standard exercise. Mean values are indicated by heights of the bars. Right side: Comparative fitness of students who elect no physical education, some physical education, or all physical education in high school: heart rate response to a standard exercise.

the physical education and band groups on the one hand and art and chorus on the other, were significant of the 5 percent level for boys but not for girls. At the time the step test was administered (over two years earlier, on the average) more than half the children were not yet in high school. This supports the hypothesis that the fitter children tend to elect physical education or band and the less fit tend to elect art or chorus when they become high school students.

Enrollment in Physical Education During High School

The official school records were consulted to determine the elective pattern chosen by each boy or girl during all years in school. The boys and girls were then grouped as to whether they had never elected physical education, had elected physical education approximately half of the semesters (seniors: 3, 4, or 5 semesters; juniors: 2, 3, or 4 semesters; sophomores: 2 semesters; freshmen, none in this category), or had elected physical education all of their high school semesters. Again, transfer students were excluded.

Fitness Tests, 1966

The three physical education groups were then compared in age-specific mean scores on the various fitness tests. The 18-year-olds were

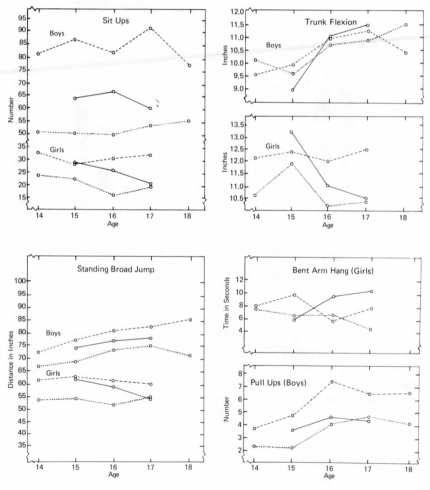

Fig. 9.2 Comparative fitness of students who elect no physical education (dotted line), some physical education (solid line), and all physical education (broken line) : situps, trunk flexion, standing broad jump, and pullups (bent-arm hang).

excluded from the analyses because in most instances their number was quite small. However, if the N was 10 or more the mean score was plotted. The results are illustrated in Figures 9.2 and 9.3. The age-specific means for the three physical education groups were compared by analysis of variance for each fitness test (Table 9.5). In this analysis the main effect reflects the significance of the differences in mean fitness scores among the three physical education groups over all ages. The interaction (groups versus age) indicated whether or not there is a difference in the slopes of the lines fitted to the scores at ages 14 through 17 (roughly freshman through senior class standing)

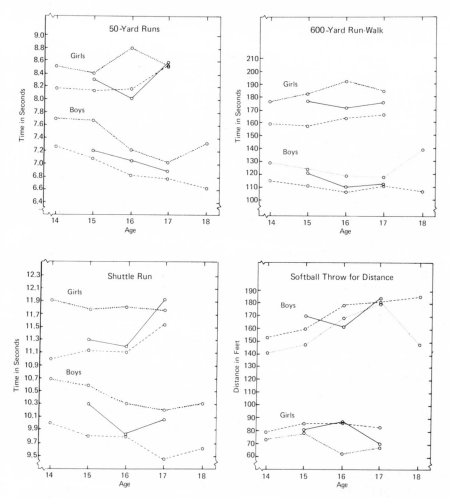

Fig. 9.3 Comparative fitness of students who elect no physical education (dotted line), some physical education (solid line), and all physical education (broken line): 50-yard run, 600-yard run-walk, shuttle run, and softball throw.

for the three groups. This is to say, it is possible to determine whether means for the three physical education groups show a significantly different relation at age 14 than at age 15, 16, or 17. From Figures 9.2 and 9.3 and Table 9.5, the pattern can be seen to be the same for boys and girls. Except for the trunk flexion and extension tests,[3] children who were enrolled in physical education all semesters scored higher in all tests. Those never enrolled in physical education scored lowest and those with some physical education were in an intermediate position. This was true across all ages (class standings). The changes with age were essentially the same in all three physical education groups.

Table 9.5

ANALYSIS OF VARIANCE: FITNESS SCORES AND AMOUNT OF PHYSICAL EDUCATION (*F*-VALUES)

	Main Effect[a] *(Amount of PE)*		*Interaction*[b] *(Age vs. Amount of PE)*	
	Boys	*Girls*	*Boys*	*Girls*
Pullups	17.52[c]	—	.75	—
Arm-Hang	—	1.95	—	1.27
Trunk Flexion	.01	8.92[c]	.72	1.23
Trunk Extension	.24	3.17[c]	.53	1.38
Shuttle Run	27.71[c]	14.82[c]	.66	1.29
Long Jump	21.21[c]	19.10[c]	.21	1.10
Situps	64.49[c]	18.41[c]	.78	1.49
50-yd Dash	19.30[c]	6.44[c]	.98	1.70
Softball Throw	3.08[c]	9.12[c]	1.64	1.48
600-yd Run-Walk	12.19[c]	14.08[c]	.39	.55

[a]*Degrees of freedom, main effects: 2; 356 for boys, 2;290 for girls.*
[b]*Degrees of freedom, interaction: 5; 356 for boys, 5; 290 for girls.*
[c]*Significant ($p < .05$).*

Step Test Results

The mean exercise heart rates for the various groups are shown in the right side of Figure 9.1. These means are adjusted for age and period between data collection. Although analysis of variance did not reveal a difference between groups, significant at the 5 percent level, the boys and girls on the average who had higher heart rates (poorer fitness) tended not to enroll in physical education.

[3]The graph for the extension test is not shown, but girls enrolled in physical education had higher scores at each age than those not enrolled in physical education. There was no consistent pattern among boys.

Conclusions

The results of the first analysis—i.e., fitness of subjects grouped by current elective, were not unexpected. Obviously one cannot be sure the superior fitness of boys and girls enrolled in physical education is due to participation in that class. Similarly, the intermediate fitness of those in band or the inferior fitness of those in art and chorus cannot with assurance be ascribed to participation in these activities. Selection may also play a role. It is logical to expect the more fit chidren and the more skilled in sports to select physical education as an elective. If this is the case, it is evident that when given a free choice, high school children will gravitate toward those activities in which they are already skilled and avoid those in which they are not.

The analysis by amount of physical education (second analysis) was planned for two reasons. First, a boy or girl might, for example, be currently enrolled in physical education but could have been enrolled in art the five previous semesters. Grouping the boys and girls who had selected physical education as an elective exclusively during their years in high school provides a more homogenous group for comparison. Second, it was thought that the second analysis would more clearly reveal the effects, if any, of participation in the physical education class.

The pattern for boys and girls was similar. The children who elected physical education as freshmen (14-year-olds) already scored significantly higher on the tests than those who elected band, art, or chorus. This is probably more a matter of the fit electing physical education. Moreover, in the other age groups when one compares those who elected physical education exclusively with those who took other subjects, about the same average difference in scores can be seen. In other words, the seniors who elected physical education exclusively are still superior to about the same degree as in the comparison of freshmen. Participation in physical education appears to have had little effect. This, of course, is a cross-sectional study. Would a longitudinal study, in which the same children are retested, show the same results? Evidence that it likely would appears in the analysis of how frequently a child elects physical education at age 14 and, in later years, elects something else. An inspection of the data revealed that among juniors and seniors, two-thirds had either never enrolled in physical education during their high school careers or had enrolled in physical education every semester. Two possibilities might be offered in the way of explanation of the lack of effect of the class in physical education. Perhaps the particular fitness tests employed might be insensitive to the changes that occurred as a result of electing or not electing physical education, or perhaps the improvement that occurred in most tests from age 14 to 17, regardless of the elective, is due to growth and/or activities that occur outside the physical education classes.

It should be pointed out that scores in the trunk flexion and extension tests are not a part of the youth fitness battery and were not as closely related to participation in physical education classes as the other scores. These two tests were included as a part of the long-range health study in this community, and not necessarily as a measure of fitness as understood in physical education.

Chapter 10 / Fitness, Fatness, and Physical Activity

Introduction

During the Renaissance period, Flemish artists often depicted plump, even corpulent women and children as ideally beautiful. Rubens was a master of this style. Even today in some parts of Europe and elsewhere it is considered a mark of beauty and health to be somewhat overly fat. In some countries of the world where starvation and diseases such as tuberculosis are serious concerns for a large part of the population, plumpness is, to some degree, an indicator of health. This does not generally apply to countries with a high standard of living. The erroneous concept perhaps arose from a mother's desire to show others that her child was well cared for and properly fed and that her "good cooking" was appreciated. It is true, of course, that if a baby or young child is not growing or gaining in weight, this is frequently a sign of impaired health. Nevertheless, evidence is lacking that plumpness in children is healthful. As a matter of fact, laboratory experiments with protozoa, flies, silkworms, rats, and cattle (134) have shown that underfeeding is more healthful and actually increases longevity.

Among adults, the association of obesity and more moderate degrees of excessive fatness with disease has been the subject of many investigations. Dr. Hundley at the National Institutes of Health (175) has summarized studies of the percentage of adults who are considerably overweight[1] and concluded that roughly

---

[1]In most cases these people are also probably overfat.

one-fifth of persons past the age of 30 are sufficiently overweight for their health to be affected. Furthermore, in males, the percentage of overweight adults has increased in recent years (279).

It is also clear that obese people, as a group, have a shorter life expectancy than the general population. A number of research papers have summarized studies that bear upon this point (7, 175, 202, 224, 225, 226, 230). Differences of opinion arise when attempting to answer such questions as: Is the increased mortality entirely due to excessive fatness or is greater muscle bulk also involved? As pointed out by Keys and Brozek (203), previous studies often have not made a careful distinction between overweight and overfat. How much excess fat must one accumulate before it becomes a health hazard? The seriousness of the problem has also been debated. For example, Dr. Edgar S. Gordon of the University of Wisconsin states:

> It is probable that no single measure would result in a more gratifying improvement in the morbidity and mortality rate from a wide variety of degenerative diseases than the obliteration of obesity as a clinical problem if it could be accomplished. (146)

On the other hand, Dr. Ancel Keys of the University of Minnesota concludes that "at best the removal of obesity in the United States would not seem to change the total adult mortality picture very much" (202). Yet all agree there is some decrease in longevity associated with obesity.

The decreased longevity associated with obesity appears to be accounted for mainly in the high death rates from cardiovascular-renal and digestive diseases, diabetes, and disorders of the liver (175, 279). However, there is a suspicion that excess fatness may be a factor in hypertension, gallbladder disease, degenerative joint disease, and certain types of cancer (202). Metabolic and chronic diseases are becoming more important as causes of death. Research is currently being directed toward the precursors of these diseases with a view to their prevention. Excessive body fatness has been implicated as a risk factor in a number of instances. To all this must be added such observations as increased surgical risk in the obese, their poor agility and hence greater proneness to injury, and feet and leg complication due to the excess weight.

Adipose or fat tissue, of course, has a useful function. It serves as an efficient method of storing fuel for metabolism. For example, in zebu (Brahman) cattle and the camel, the hump serves as a store of reserve fat and shows seasonal changes depending on the food supply (45). Salmon, when returning to spawn, are able to swim great distances while utilizing stored fat for energy. Some birds, before migration, store fat in a special organ from which they draw energy during the long flight (267). Subcutaneous fat also serves as insulation and has a certain aesthetic function when deposited in optimum amounts and when distributed properly. There are some activities in which fatness is not a handicap. In synchronized swimming, the higher percentage of fat in girls and consequently their greater buoyancy likely contribute to a smoother performance in some maneuvers.

The Measurement of Body Fatness

There have been exceller symposia on the measurement of body composition in recent years (35, 46, 47), but the article by Keys and Brozek (203) remains as one of the best discussions of body composition and the measurement of body fatness. The human or animal body may be thought of as being composed of four major substances, namely: (a) bone, (b) water, (c) fat, and (d) muscles and internal organs. With regard to the measurement of body fatness, variations in bone density is of minor significance. Even the change in bone density associated with aging does not introduce a serious error, particularly in analyses of the Tecumseh data which is generally studied within age groups. Alterations in body fluids deserve more consideration, but even the influence of this factor does not present serious difficulties in the majority of instances. Therefore, except for cases of edema, which were excluded in our analyses, normal body hydration and bone density were assumed and the assessment of body composition then became a problem of estimating the relative percentage of fat and muscle.

In recent years a number of laboratory methods of assessing body fatness have been used. These include hydrostatic weighing; estimating fat under the skin by ultrasonics; estimating body volume by air displacement, helium dilution, or by photogrammetry; creatinine excretion; estimating body potassium; and determining total body water. Despite the established validity for some of these methods, they are not practical in population studies.

Skinfolds

It is possible to grasp, between the thumb and index finger, the loose tissue over the abdomen, at the waistline or at other places on the body. This "pinch" of tissue is known as a "skinfold" and includes a double layer of skin plus subcustaneous fat. The thickness of the fold reflects the amount of fat under the skin and is measured in millimeters with a "skinfold caliper."

The measurement of skinfold thickness is not a difficult procedure. However, several precautions are necessary. The procedure must be standardized with regard to (a) the site on the body where the skinfold is to be taken and (b) the distance from the point at which the skinfold is lifted and the site at which the calipers are applied.[2] When pressure is applied with the

[2]This is important because the skinfold should be compressed by the calipers, not by the experimenter's fingers.

calipers, the thickness of the skinfold will gradually decrease because tissue is squeezed out from under the jaws of the calipers. This was thought to be a crucial source of error until Lewis and colleagues (218) demonstrated that after two seconds essentially all compression has taken place and the measurement is stabilized, except in cases of edema. Therefore, if the reading is made between about two and five seconds, little error from this source will arise.

The validity of skinfold measurements for estimating body fatness has been reviewed elsewhere (241). It has been observed (203) that the skinfold measurements of various sites on the same subjects are highly correlated ($r = .742$ to $.938$). We've observed much the same result in the Tecumseh Community Health Study, in which the correlation coefficients between triceps and subscapular skinfolds range between 0.6 and 0.8 for 10-year age groups among males and females. When the sum of four skinfolds was correlated with the sum of two, the coefficients were generally near 0.9. This means that the law of diminishing returns applies very soon and determining a few skinfolds is about as good as taking measurements at many sites. There have been numerous attempts to develop multiple regression equations based on several skinfolds and in some cases also body girths or diameters. Evidence is not clear as yet that these equations give better results than individual skinfold thickness or the sum of several skinfolds.

In the Tecumseh study during the first series of examinations, skinfolds at two sites, triceps and subscapular, were measured by means of the C-caliper developed at the Laboratory of Physiological Hygiene, University of Minnesota. The calipers were calibrated by suspending a known weight on one of the jaws and adjusting the spring until the force exerted was 10 gm per sq mm. In the second and third series of examinations in Tecumseh, a Lange caliper was used and two more sites, abdomen and waist, were added. The calibration of the Lange calipers was determined by means of small springs with known force-compression curves.

The measurements were taken as follows:

TRICEPS SKINFOLD. This measurement is taken at a site halfway between the tip of the acromial process and tip of the elbow. The arm should be hanging freely. The skinfold is lifted on the back of the right arm parallel to long axis of the arm about 1 cm above the site. Calipers are allowed to compress skinfold about 1 cm below the point where the skinfold is lifted (Figure 10.1 A).

SUBSCAPULAR SKINFOLD. The skinfold is lifted at the tip of the right scapula on a diagonal plane about 45° from the horizontal (laterally downward). The calipers are used about 1 cm laterally downward from this point (Figure 10.1 B).

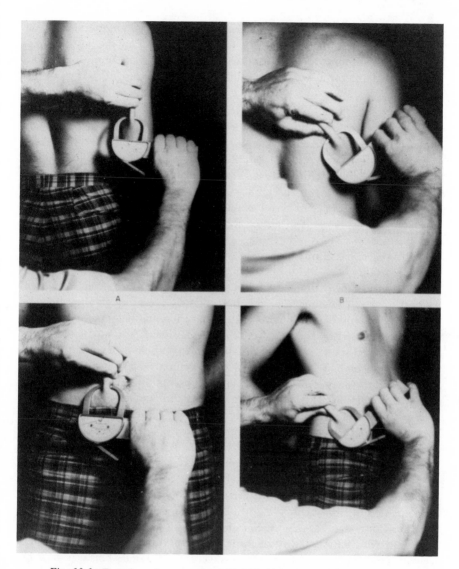

Fig. 10.1 Technique for measuring skinfold thickness. A, Triceps; B. Subscapular; C. Abdominal; and D. Waist. Reproduced from (241) with permission of the publisher.

ABDOMINAL SKINFOLD. The skinfold is lifted about 1 cm to the right of the umbilicus and parallel to the long axis of the body. The calipers are held so that the jaws are vertical about 1 cm below the point at which the skinfold is lifted (Figure 10.1 C).

WAIST SKINFOLD. The skinfold is lifted on the right mid-axillary line just above the crest of the ilium. The fold is lifted to follow the natural diagonal line at this point (dorsally upward). The calipers are again used about 1 cm from the point at which the skinfold is lifted (Figure 10.1 D).

Relative Weight

Most, if not all, readers are familiar with the age-height-weight tables for males and females which were developed by insurance company statisticians. Each value in these tables is an "average" weight for a given age, sex, and height. This value is not necessarily an ideal weight but rather the average weight for people of a particular sex, age, and height who are examined for insurance. There have also been extensive tables compiled as a result of measurements of armed forces personnel and in other state and national surveys. More recently tables of "ideal" or desirable weights have been compiled based on the weight for a given height associated with the lowest mortality.

It is well-known that people who are muscular and stocky are overweight by these "average" or "ideal" standards even though they may be lean. Welham and Behnke demonstrated that the usual height-age-sex tables are inadequate when they showed that professional football players were rated very much overweight by the tables and yet these men were quite lean as determined by body specific gravity measurements (365). Keys and Brozek (204) raised the question whether or not such exceptions are common enough to warrant concern. They classified people by the age-height-sex tables and also by more refined methods of measuring body fatness. It was clear that if one wishes to categorize people by body fatness, a large percentage of subjects are misclassified by such insurance company tables.

More recently, insurance company tables have included mean values based on three body builds: small, medium, and large frame (203). However, because no objective criteria are provided for classifying body builds, this refinement is of little help. Weight is likely more closely related to volume than to a linear measurement such as height. This has produced a number of studies in which the validity of insurance tables and ratios of height and weight as measures of total body fatness were investigated. This was done by comparing estimates of fatness utilizing a laboratory method with the degree a subject is over- and underweight according to the insurance or a height-weight table. These studies are reviewed elsewhere (241). Various height-weight ratios are not much better than insurance tables based on height alone.

Some people are reluctant to accept the validity of skinfolds. Also, it is inconvenient, and sometimes impossible, to estimate from skinfolds the degree of obesity in pounds. Therefore, a "relative weight" index was also calculated for the Tecumseh respondents. The procedures have been published elsewhere (241, 247). This index is likely less accurate than skinfolds for estimating body fatness.

Relation of Fatness to Habitual Physical Activity

In most cases, the amount of fat accumulated is the result of a simple equation which includes food intake (calories) on the one hand and energy expenditure (calories) on the other. If a person who is in caloric balance increases food intake without changing energy expenditure, fat will accumulate. But fat will also accumulate if the food intake is held constant and energy expenditure is decreased. This is well-known to the farmer who

Table 10.1

BODY FATNESS (SUM OF FOUR SKINFOLDS) AND
HABITUAL PHYSICAL ACTIVITY
(ALL SUBJECTS)

Physical Activity Index	*Groups Compared*	*Mean Sum of Skinfolds*	*N*	*Age Groups Where Difference in Means is Significant, $p < .05$*
Mean	Highest	83.6	275	Over all Ages
WMR/BMR	Intermediate	86.7	818	
Occ. + Leisure	Lowest	92.3	273	35–44
Mean	Highest	83.3	445	Over all Ages
WMR/BMR	Intermediate	89.0	647	
Occ. Only	Lowest	89.3	274	
Hours	Most	89.0	273	25–34
Occ. Only	Intermediate	89.0	398	
	Least	85.4	695	45–54
Active	Highest	87.4	281	
Leisure	Intermediate	86.6	800	
Index	Lowest	88.7	285	
Mean WMR/BMR	Highest	86.7	273	
Active Leisure	Intermediate	87.9	838	
Only	Lowest	85.3	255	
Hours	Most	87.0	273	
Active Leisure	Intermediate	87.3	819	
Only	Least	87.1	274	
	Farmers	81.4	181	

Reproduced from (254) with permission of the publisher.

"pens up" animals to fatten them. One would expect, therefore, a correlation between fatness and sedentary living. However, differences in groups are becoming more difficult to demonstrate because labor-saving devices have reduced the physical exercise in even the blue-collar jobs, and their work day is shorter. Also, a rise in the standard of living in the United States has made calories in almost any form more readily available to workers—including manual laborers.

It is abundantly clear that obese children are less active then children of normal weight, the former having a history of infrequent participation in sports. This observation has been repeated a number of times, both here and abroad. The studies are reviewed elsewhere (230, 231, 232, 278). It is obvious that a vicious cycle develops in which reduced activity results in increased fatness which, in turn, results in further reduction in activity. However, there is evidence that a decrease in physical activity precedes and is responsible for triggering this cycle in many adolescents (231).

Table 10.1 shows a comparison of the sum of four skinfolds in Tecumseh males grouped by habitual physical activity by the methods described in Chapter 3. Mean energy expenditure for occupational activity (Mean WMR/BMR, occupation only) was significantly related to body fatness but the relationship is strengthened if leisure activity is also included. Leisure activity alone was not significantly related to the sum of four skinfolds. Farmers were the leanest group, on the average.

Relative weight showed similar trends but the relationships with habitual physical activity were not as close as for sum of skinfolds.

Relation of Fatness to Physical Fitness and Enrollment in Physical Education

Body fatness (sum of four skinfolds) was compared in boys and girls who select various electives in high school. Because the skinfold measurements were taken from 9 to 47 months earlier, they were corrected for (a) age and (b) time between measurement and assessment of high school elective. The adjusted means for boys and girls enrolled in physical education, band, chorus, or art are shown in Figure 10.2 (left panel). Analysis of covariance revealed that the difference in means was significant for boys but not for girls. Further analysis using the Duncan Multiple Range Test indicated that the band and physical education groups were similar but both were different from the art and chorus groups, which were in turn similar to each other.

On the right side of Figure 10.2 is shown a similar comparison, but in this instance the children were grouped as to whether they elected physical education all semesters, some semesters, or never elected physical education in high school. Again the differences were statistically significant for boys but not for girls. From the results of Figure 10.2, it appears clear that in the case of boys, those children who are fatter, given a choice, generally do not elect physical education when they reach high school. This tendency was detectable in girls but the results were not statistically significant.

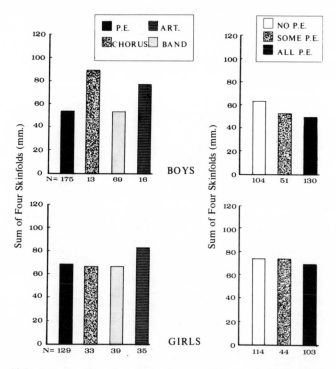

Fig. 10.2 Left side: The relationship of current high school elective and body fatness (sum of skinfolds). Mean values are indicated by height of bars. Right side: Comparative fatness of students who elect no physical education, some physical education, or all physical education in high school.

Age- and sex-specific correlation coefficients between the physical fitness tests (Chapter 9) and sum of skinfolds are shown in Table 10.2. In these correlations, the effects of (a) interval between skinfold measurements and physical fitness test, (b) height, and (c) weight were removed by partial correlation. Statistically significant coefficients ($p < .05$) are denoted with an asterisk. From the many significant correlation coefficients, it is clear that children who are relatively fatter do poorer in most fitness tests, even though fitness was measured, on the average, 26 months later.

Table 10.2 PARTIAL CORRELATION COEFFICIENTS: SUM OF FOUR SKINFOLDS VS. AAHPER YOUTH FITNESS SCORES (EFFECTS OF HEIGHT, WEIGHT AND INTERVAL BETWEEN TESTS REMOVED)

Fitness Test	Age									
	9	10	11	12	13	14	15	16	17	18
Boys										
Pullups	.22	.01	.02	-.28*	-.27*	-.29*	-.20	-.31*	-.32*	-.31*
Long Jump	-.22	-.07	-.08	-.32*	-.37*	-.14	-.42*	-.22	-.22	-.46*
Speed in Shuttle Run	.02	.16	-.13	-.40*	-.29*	-.14	-.32*	-.42*	-.42*	-.54*
Situps	.00	-.22*	-.08	-.29*	-.18	-.11	-.13	-.30*	-.13	-.21
Speed in 50-yd Run	-.03	-.02	-.26*	-.40*	-.31*	-.08	-.39*	-.41*	-.31*	-.42*
Softball Throw	-.06	-.11	-.19	-.35*	-.26*	-.08	-.24*	-.41*	0.01	-.35
Speed in 600-yd Run	.20	-.07	-.12	-.29*	-.32*	-.17	-.41*	-.37*	-.30*	-.24
N=	50	88–89	100–102	102–106	90–93	86–91	80–87	72–77	66–72	31–34
Girls										
Arm-Hang	-.14	-.18	-.16	-.11	-.16	-.15	-.06	-.19	-.09	-.33
Long Jump	-.16	-.34*	-.21	-.01	.05	-.30*	-.08	-.24	-.26	-.16
Speed in Shuttle Run	.01	-.26*	-.28*	.06	-.01	-.27*	-.22	-.28*	-.25	-.30
Situps	-.21	-.21	-.22	.11	-.13	-.29*	-.02	-.11	-.12	.01
Speed in 50-yd Run	-.15	-.38*	-.28*	-.15	-.18	-.23*	-.27*	-.35*	-.22	.23
Softball Throw	-.07	-.21	-.14	-.13	-.04	-.28*	-.04	-.03	.09	-.60
Speed in 600-yd Run	-.21	-.35*	-.15	-.24*	-.17	-.26*	.02	-.35*	.04	-.13
N=	55	80–82	81–86	87	73–78	77–85	74–75	59–68	36–52	14–19

*Statistically significant, $p < 0.05$.

Chapter 11 / **Blood Pressure**

Hypertension, or high blood pressure, is related to the development of atherosclerosis and coronary heart disease (119). It is also accepted that high blood pressure has no single cause but rather results from the interaction of a number of factors (118). These likely include obesity, tension or stress, heredity, salt intake and, perhaps, sedentary living.

Average systolic and diastolic blood pressure is known to increase with age in highly developed countries, but in certain more primitive societies this is not true (118). The question may be raised whether sedentary living in the more advanced countries contributes directly or indirectly to the increase in blood pressure with age.

Habitual Physical Activity and Blood Pressure

The data reported in this section were collected in the second series of examinations in Tecumseh. Several blood pressure recordings were made. Systolic and diastolic (5th phase) blood pressure as recorded by a trained technician prior to the medical examination were used for the present analysis. Pressures were taken in the right arm with the subject in a sitting position. Habitual physical activity was assessed by the methods described in Chapter 3. Activity data were collected only on males.

The principal statistical analysis employed was a one-way analysis of variance comparing the mean blood pressure of each of the three activity groups (least active, intermediate, and most active). Systolic and diastolic blood pressure increase with age in Tecumseh (181), as is true of most populations in the United States. Hence in order to eliminate the effects of age, the variance analyses were done in age-specific groups and then combined over all ages. Data on farmers were not included in the statistical analysis because it was not possible to calculate physical activity indices for this group. The mean values for the farmers are included for comparison.

Detailed results are reported elsewhere (254), but the most important findings are summarized below. Tables 11.1 and 11.2 show a comparison of the physical activity groups by systolic and diastolic pressure. In these and subsequent similar tables, only those age groups are indicated in which statistical significance at the 5 percent level was reached. It can be seen that the least active men, classified on the basis of estimates of total energy expenditure (occupation and leisure), had the highest mean blood pressures, both systolic and diastolic. Within each of the specific age groups shown,

Table 11.1

SYSTOLIC BLOOD PRESSURE AND HABITUAL PHYSICAL ACTIVITY
(ALL SUBJECTS)

Physical Activity Index	Groups Compared	Mean SBP	N	Age Groups Where Difference in Means is Significant, $p < .05$*
Mean	Highest	137.3	275	35–44
WMR/BMR	Intermediate	137.9	816	
Occ. + Leisure	Lowest	140.4	270	45–54
Mean	Highest	137.8	445	35–44
WMR/BMR	Intermediate	137.9	645	
Occ. Only	Lowest	140.0	271	
Hours	Most	139.5	273	25–34
Occ. Only	Intermediate	138.6	397	
	Least	137.6	691	
Active	Highest	137.5	280	
Leisure	Intermediate	138.3	797	
Index	Lowest	139.9	284	
Mean WMR/BMR	Highest	136.5	255	45–54
Active Leisure	Intermediate	138.5	834	
Only	Lowest	139.4	255	
Hours	Most	139.5	273	
Active Leisure	Intermediate	138.5	816	
Only	Least	138.3	272	
	Farmers	138.2	179	

*Only the age groups showing an F-value with a probability less than .05 are shown.
Reproduced from (254) with permission of the publisher.

Table 11.2

DIASTOLIC BLOOD PRESSURE AND HABITUAL PHYSICAL ACTIVITY
(ALL SUBJECTS)

Physical Activity Index	Groups Compared	Mean DBP	N	Age Groups Where Difference in Means is Significant, p < .05*
Mean	Highest	77.9	274	Over All Ages
WMR/BMR	Intermediate	78.5	815	
Occ. + Leisure	Lowest	80.8	270	45–54
Mean	Highest	78.5	445	Over All Ages
WMR/BMR	Intermediate	78.2	643	
Occ. Only	Lowest	80.9	271	45–54
Hours	Most	78.8	272	
Occupation	Intermediate	78.7	397	
Only	Least	79.0	690	
Active	Highest	78.3	279	
Leisure	Intermediate	78.8	796	
Index	Lowest	79.2	284	
Mean WMR/BMR	Highest	78.2	272	
Active	Intermediate	78.8	832	
Leisure Only	Lowest	79.6	255	
Hours	Most	78.6	272	
Active	Intermediate	78.9	815	
Leisure Only	Least	78.7	272	
	Farmers	78.1	179	

*Only the age groups showing an F-value with a probability less than .05 are shown.
Reproduced from (254) with permission of the publisher.

the mean blood pressure was highest in the least active and lowest in the most active, as was also true for all ages combined (column 3 in Tables 11.1 and 11.2).

This was also true when the respondents were classified on the basis of average energy expenditure in *occupation only*. However, when subjects were classified on the basis of hours worked per week, the men who worked the most hours had the highest mean systolic blood pressure, which was not quite significant over all ages but reached significance in age group 25 to 34. It was considered possible that the men who worked the longer hours were those in the sedentary occupations (professional, managerial, clerks, etc.) and hence the relationship between hours worked and blood pressure might be only a reflection of the lower rate of energy expenditure during work. However, a closer look at the data revealed that the men who worked the longest hours were not primarily those with the sedentary jobs. Thus the tendency for higher blood pressure in men who worked the longest hours was not explained by a lower rate of energy expenditure in their occupations.

The trend for higher blood pressures among men expending less energy in their leisure time is detectable but not statistically significant in most cases. It is understandable that occupation, generally involving eight or more hours per day, might overshadow any effect of leisure activity. Therefore, the analysis for leisure activity was repeated in those men who were classified as least active in their occupation. There was no statistically significant difference in blood pressures among these subjects classified on the basis of their active leisure activities.

It was thought to be of interest to study the leisure activity of only those who worked the longest hours (more than 50 hours per week). The analysis indicated a tendency for the men who spend more hours and total energy in active leisure to have lower diastolic blood pressure (statistically significant in ages 20 to 44). However, this was not true with regard to systolic blood pressure.

Influence of Body Fatness

It is well-known that a correlation exists between body fatness and blood pressure in most populations (63). Table 11.3 indicates this is

Table 11.3

CORRELATION OF SUM OF FOUR SKINFOLDS WITH SYSTOLIC
AND DIASTOLIC BLOOD PRESSURE

| | *Correlation Coefficients* | | |
Age Group	*SBP*	*DBP*	*N*
16–19	.562*	.225	29
20–24	.429*	.223*	117
25–34	.260*	.315*	390
35–44	.278*	.352*	480
45–54	.190*	.184*	312
55–64	.163*	.359*	179

*Significant, $p < .05$
Reproduced from (254) with permission of the publisher.

also true of our Tecumseh male subjects for whom we had physical activity data. It is interesting to note that the correlation of systolic blood pressure with fatness decreases with age. As pointed out in Chapter 10, the more active subjects are also leaner. This was especially true when both occupation and leisure activities were used to classify the men. The question may then be raised: Is the higher blood pressure in the least active men due to the greater fatness of these subjects? In order to look into this question further, the respondents within each age category were grouped by the sum of four skinfolds (triceps, subscapular, umbilical, and suprailiac) such that the one-third with the largest skinfolds were together (upper third); the one-third with lowest sum of skinfolds were combined similarly (lower third); and the rest formed the "middle third" group. Within each of these body fatness groups, the mean systolic and diastolic blood pressures were compared among the three physical activity groups (based on mean WMR/BMR for occupation and leisure). The results appear in Tables 11.4 and 11.5. The numbers in each subgroup

Table 11.4

SYSTOLIC BLOOD PRESSURE AND HABITUAL PHYSICAL ACTIVITY
(MEAN WMR/BMR, OCCUPATION AND LEISURE)
IN THREE BODY FATNESS GROUPS

Physical Activity Group *Mean WMR/BMR* *Occupation and Leisure*	*Body Fatness Group (Sum of 4 Skinfolds)*					
	Upper Third *Mean* *SBP*	*N*	*Middle Third* *Mean* *SBP*	*N*	*Lower Third* *Mean* *SBP*	*N*
Highest	140.2	82	140.5	91	132.0	102
Intermediate	141.8	285	137.6	262	134.0	269
Lowest	143.4	104	138.8	98	138.3	68
Age Groups Where Difference in Means is Significant, $p < .05$			20–24		Over all Ages	
Farmers	141.7	56	140.8	56	133.1	67

Reproduced from (254) with permission of the publisher.

Table 11.5

DIASTOLIC BLOOD PRESSURE AND HABITUAL PHYSICAL ACTIVITY
(MEAN WMR/BMR, OCCUPATION AND LEISURE)
IN THREE BODY FATNESS GROUPS

Physical Activity Group *Mean WMR/BMR* *Occupation and Leisure*	*Body Fatness Group (Sum of 4 Skinfolds)*					
	Upper Third *Mean* *DBP*	*N*	*Middle Third* *Mean* *DBP*	*N*	*Lower Third* *Mean* *DBP*	*N*
Highest	82.0	81	79.7	91	73.1	102
Intermediate	81.8	284	79.2	262	74.2	269
Lowest	83.4	104	79.5	98	78.6	68
Age Groups Where Difference in Means is Significant, $p < .05$					Over all Ages	
Farmers	80.1	56	79.9	56	74.9	67

Reproduced from (254) with permission of the publisher.

become small; hence it is more difficult to demonstrate statistical significance. The trend is for higher blood pressures to be associated with the least physical activity, but the association is statistically significant only among the leanest subjects. In all three activity groups and among the farmers as well, the higher blood pressures are found among the fattest subjects. It appears that the independent contribution of fatness to blood pressure may be greater than the contribution of inactivity but the largest gradients in both Tables 11.4 and 11.5 are from the most active, leanest subjects to the least active, fattest ones.

Influence of Smoking Habits

The relation between blood pressure and physical activity may be further confounded by smoking habits. In our data there was no significant relationship of systolic blood pressure to smoking habits, but male cigarette smokers tended to have slightly but significantly lower diastolic pressure. This has been reported previously in the Tecumseh data (166). There appeared to be little or no relationship between physical activity and smoking habits except that there were more nonsmokers among the farmers. Therefore, smoking habits likely could not explain or obscure the relationship between physical activity and blood pressure. Nevertheless, the subjects were grouped by smoking habits. Blood pressure was then studied in relation to physical activity within each smoking group, as was done for body fatness. In all smoking groups, the highest mean systolic and diastolic blood pressure was found in the least active group.

Discussion

The increase in blood pressure with age which is characteristic of people in more highly developed societies is not seen in many primitive populations (118). Primitive people are invariably more active and leaner and, at least in the Kalahari Bushmen (187), there is no correlation between blood pressure and weight-height ratio.

In a number of previous studies, physical activity (primarily of occupation) has been studied in relation to blood pressure. These investigations are summarized in Table 11.6. In addition, Chrastek and co-workers (65) quoted two Russian reports that the frequency of hypertension is lower among people whose occupations require manual labor as compared to white-collar workers. This summary (Table 11.6) reveals that all population studies are not consistent. However, except for one study (174), where a difference exists, the lower blood pressures are found in the more active workers. Also body fatness is generally lower in these subjects.

Taylor (351) made the interesting observation that the active switchmen in his study of railroad personnel did not have different blood pressures from

Table 11.6

COMPARISON OF ACTIVE AND INACTIVE POPULATIONS IN RESTING BLOOD PRESSURE AND BODY FATNESS: REVIEW OF PREVIOUS STUDIES

Groups Compared	Systolic BP	Diastolic BP	Body Fatness	Reference
377 athletes, 652 nonathletes				
Normal weight	Athletes, lower	Athletes, lower	—	Anderson and Elvik, 1956 (6)
Overweight	Athletes, lower	Athletes, lower	—	
1,045 men, age 60–69	No diff.	No diff.	Not compared	Brown et al., 1956 (44)
1,860 men, various occupations	Heavy workers, higher	Not compared	Not compared	Humerfelt and Wederwang, 1957 (174)
60 heavy workers, 180 light workers	Heavy workers, lower	Heavy workers, lower	Not compared	Miall and Oldham, 1958 (237)
3,000 noncoronary deaths	Active, less hypertension		Not compared	Morris and Crawford, 1958 (262, p. 177, 263)
1,360 Chicago utility company workers	No diff.	No diff.	No. diff.	Berkson et al., 1960 (23)
852 London transportation and other workers	Active, lower	Active, lower	Active, leaner	Morris, 1960 (261, 262, p. 177)
369 Finnish lumberjacks and 421 less active men	Lumberjack, lower	Lumberjack, lower	Not compared	Karvonen et al., 1961 (195)
20 active ama (Korean divers) and 20 controls	Ama, lower	No diff.	Not compared	Kang et al., 1963 (188)
29 active and 79 inactive professional men	No diff.	No diff.	Not compared	Raab and Krzywanek, 1965 (297)
114 active and 111 inactive YMCA members	No diff.	No diff.	No diff.	Doan et al., 1965 (103), 1966 (104)
Men, aged 40–59 in seven countries	Active, lower	Active, lower	Active, leaner	Keys et al., 1967 (205)
5,127 males and females, age 37–72	No diff.	Not reported	Not reported	Dauber et al., 1967 (92)
416 active and 298 less active RR workers	Active, lower	No diff.	Active, leaner	Taylor, 1967 (351) and Keys et al., 1967 (205)
100 pedicabmen and 1,346 less active Chinese	No diff.	No diff.	Active, leaner	Chiang et al., 1968 (60)
247 healthy males, age 40–50	No diff.	No diff.	Active, leaner	Schwalb, 1968 (325)
8,948 civil servants, grouped by distance walked to work	No diff.	Not compared	Active, leaner	Rose, 1969 (317)
30 active and 26 sedentary middle-aged men	No diff.	Active, lower	Not compared	Whitsett and Naughton, 1971 (373)

the less active clerks when starting their employment, but the active group had lower pressures later in life. This suggests that the differences were not due to selection. Miall and Oldham (237) (Table 11.6) adjusted their comparison of blood pressure of workers in light and heavy occupations for upper-arm girth and the lower blood pressures in the more active subjects persisted. They also showed that a difference in social class could not account for the difference in blood pressure. Kapeller-She (189) reported that among 111 persons who had engaged in regular physical activity for a long time only about 25 percent showed evidence of being "prehypertensive" (standard cold test), whereas 42 percent of 265 sedentary subjects showed this tendency. Thomas (361) reported results similar to ours regarding the higher blood pressures among men working longer hours.

In summary, most studies, including our own, indicate that active men have lower blood pressures than more sedentary people. In most previous studies, the numbers of cases have been too small to isolate the relationship of physical activity to blood pressure from the relationship of body fatness to blood pressures. From our analysis, physical activity and body fatness

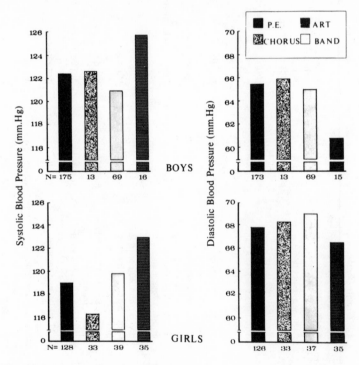

Fig. 11.1 The relationship of current high school elective and blood pressure. Mean values are indicated by height of bars.

are independently related to blood pressure, the former inversely and the latter directly.

The small absolute differences in blood pressure among activity groups, although statistically significant, may appear unimportant. However, Cornfield (76) has pointed out that 1 percent difference in systolic blood pressure at the lower range is associated with a 4.6 percent difference in risk of coronary heart disease and a 2.6 percent difference in risk in coronary heart disease at the upper range. Furthermore, the difficulties in classifying large numbers of people by energy expenditures are well-known. The methods, including ours, are crude and it is possible that some of our subjects are misclassified. There are also problems with obtaining accurate blood pressure measurements. Additionally, there are surely subjects in all three groups with hypertension from causes unrelated to physical activity. Finally, the range in physical activity is not great because only a small percentage of people in the United States are physically active. All of these factors tend to reduce the blood pressure gradient by physical activity. Despite all this, men who are less active have been shown to have higher blood pressures, both systolic and diastolic. Occupation alone shows this phenomenon, but the relationship is strengthened if leisure activities are also considered.

Relation to Physical Fitness and Enrollment in Physical Education

As described in Chapter 9, measurements, including blood pressure, were taken in the laboratory on many of the children in the Tecumseh School System. On the average, 26 months later, the physical fitness of these children was measured and for those in high school their pattern of elective was determined. The blood pressure data were corrected for age and months since physical fitness testing.

Figure 11.1 shows the adjusted mean blood pressure, for high school students selecting various electives. The differences in means were not statistically significant for boys or girls. When the students were grouped by how consistently they elected physical education in high school, there likewise were not statistically significant differences in the means (Figure 11.2).

Age- and sex-specific correlation coefficients were calculated between systolic and diastolic blood pressure and the physical fitness tests described in Chapter 9. Except for an occasional significant coefficient, probably due to chance, blood pressure was unrelated to the physical fitness scores even when the effects of height and weight were removed.

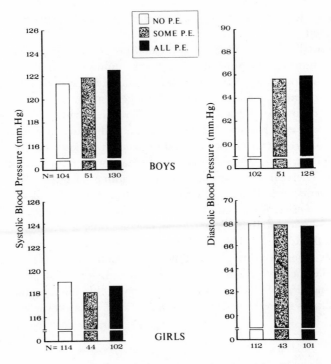

Fig. 11.2 Systolic and diastolic blood pressure of students who elect no physical education, some physical education, or all physical education in high school. Mean values are indicated by height of bars.

Chapter **12** / **Cardiac Pre-ejection Period**

It may not be readily apparent why cardiac pre-ejection period was measured in the Tecumseh population. A brief introductory discussion will be given to provide the rationale.

Stress and Heart Attacks

It is commonly believed that stresses of various kinds predispose some individuals to myocardial infarction (heart attack). This could be an acute effect that precipitates the attack or chronic exposure to stress that contributes to the chain of events leading to myocardial infarction.

Acute Stress

Many clinicians intuitively feel that an acute stress is responsible for bringing on a heart attack in some of their patients, but it is often not easy to document the sequence of events preceding the attack. Reactions to stress certainly involve the automatic nervous system (sympathetic and parasympathetic), the pituitary and the adrenal glands. Although the cortex (outer portion) of the adrenal gland secretes a number of steriods that are related to stress reactions, it is epinephrine (adrenaline), secreted from the medulla (inner portion of the gland), and perhaps norepinephrine, that have been most commonly studied in relation to stress and heart attacks. Epinephrine and norepinephrine (a closely related substance secreted mostly at the sympathetic nerve endings) are collectively referred to as catecholamines. Stresses of various kinds elicit a marked increase in catecholamine secretion. Cardiac damage has been produced in a number of species of animals by various stressors, infusion of catecholamines, and stimulation of sympathetic nerves to the heart (292). It has been suggested that the relationship between smoking and heart disease is at least partially explained by the increase in catecholamine secretion produced by nicotine. For over thirty years it has been known that changes in the electrocardiogram suggestive of inadequate blood supply to the heart may occur during states of anxiety and in other stressful situations (211, 330). When human subjects were examined shortly after death from myocardial infarction, there were differences in myocardial catecholamine concentrations as compared to people dying from other causes (296). However, this does not indicate whether these changes were the cause or result of the infarction.

After myocardial infarction, surviving patients exhibit an increase in circulating catecholamines (309, 342), as do dogs after experimentally induced occlusion of coronary arteries (309, 310). Patients with angina pectoris show abnormal increases in circulating catecholamines during excitement or as a result of standard submaximal exercise (310). Further evidence that stress might be associated with myocardial infarction is the observation that among 42 tax accountants, blood clotting time was shortened when their occupation became more stressful at certain times of the year (318).

This brief review was presented only to illustrate that there are both clinical observations and experimental data on man and animals suggesting that acute stressful situations may precipitate a heart attack.

Chronic Stress

The question of chronic effects of stress has also been of interest. Roseman and Friedman have approached this question using the interview method and have identified the "A" type, who appears to be under considerable occupational stress much of the time and who is more likely to develop clinical evidence of coronary heart disease. This type also has a higher serum concentration of cholesterol, triglyceride, and beta-lipoprotein (318). This approach identifies a personality type and this may be a more important factor than the particular chronic occupational stress involved. In any case, a quantitative biological measurement of an individual's reactivity to stress would be a useful research tool and is badly needed. Occupational stress increases catecholamine concentration in the urine (215), whereas a low level of urinary catecholamines has been observed in tranquil-living Somali herdsmen (211). However, no difference in resting catecholamine excretion was observed in active compared to sedentary young men; nor was there an effect of twelve weeks of training on resting catecholamine excretion (350). There are technical difficulties in such studies so the results are not conclusive. In any case, in large epidemiologic studies, analyses of this kind have not been feasible. Also, there is a question of how closely urine concentrations of catecholamines reflect the concentrations in the blood or myocardium. Furthermore, it may be the turnover rate of catecholamines, not the concentration, that is important. Other methods must be found for use in epidemiologic investigations.

Coronary Heart Disease and Habitual Physical Activity

Space does not permit a comprehensive review of the relationship of physical activity to heart disease. It should be pointed out, however, that most of the evidence comes from epidemiologic studies dating back to about 1939 in which mortality rates of various occupational groups have been studied. In over twenty such studies, the age-specific mortality from heart disease, with one exception, has been higher among men in the more sedentary occupations. The evidence that physical activity alters the development or course of atherosclerosis is not impressive. However, it appears that people who are more active can tolerate coronary atherosclerosis better than those who are less active. Whether this is due to greater collateral circulation in the heart, changes in clotting or lysis time, less sympathetic stimulation, or some other mechanisms, is not known.

Habitual Physical Activity and Stress

It remains to be seen whether the concentration of catecholamines in the myocardium, blood, or urine of more active or athletically conditioned people is different from that of less active persons. Results with animals have been conflicting. In two studies with rats, physical conditioning (exercise) decreased catecholamine concentration in the myocardium (96, 133). On the other hand, one investigation showed an increase (280) and two others (213, 281) no change in norepinephrine in the myocardium as a result of training. Hearts hypertrophied as a result of aortic constriction had lower concentrations of norepinephrine (127).

In one rat study (301, 302) and one in dogs (192), exercise training had no effect on plasma catecholamine concentration, and in cockerels the concentration was increased (313). In still another study with rats, moderate daily exercise had no effect but exhaustive daily exercise raised plasma catecholamine concentration (64). Saltzman and colleagues (323) demonstrated that voluntary exercise in mice did not change the total uptake of epinephrine by the myocardium but that such exercise made the hearts of animals more sensitive to high doses of injected epinephrine in that more heart damage resulted (322). This supported an earlier observation in hypertrophied hearts (378). It appears that further investigations are required to clarify the effects of training on catecholamine concentration, binding capacity, and turnover in the myocardium and their relationship to stress and heart disease.

Selye (328) has reported beneficial effects of regular exercise in rats. In one series of experiments, he stressed the animals by injecting sodium acetate plus fluorocortisol. Some of the animals were conditioned to regular physical activity. All the animals were then subjected to an exhaustive bout of exercise. Exercise conditioning prevented the cardiac necrosis (myocardial infarction) that developed in the inactive animals. In another group of rats, cardiac damage was caused by electrolyte-steroid injections. Some of the animals again were conditioned with regular exercise. Bone fracture then produced cardiac necrosis in the unexercised animals but not in those exposed to regular exercise.

Cardiac Pre-ejection Period

When the ventricle is stimulated, some time is required for the electrical impulse to travel through the intraventricular conduction system and the myocardium. Another period of time lapses while tension develops in the myocardium before blood is ejected. Finally, blood is ejected until the pulmonary and aortic semilunar valves close. The time required for these events can be accurately measured with catheters in the heart but it can also be estimated by simply recording the electrocardiogram, heart sounds (phonocardiogram), and the carotid pulse wave. This is shown in the diagram (Figure 12.1) by Raab (294). The time of ventricular systole, TS in Figure 12.1, begins with the Q-wave of the ECG and terminates with the second heart sound. The more common designation for this time period is QS_2. The time during which blood is ejected from the left ventricle may be determined from the duration of the carotid pulse measured from the thinning, at the beginning of the steep systolic ascent to the dicrotic notch (see Figure 12.1). This is designated EP in the diagram but is usually referred to as the left ventricular ejection time (LVET). If the time required for left ventricular ejection is subtracted from the total time of ventricular systole, the pre-ejection period (PEP), denoted in the diagram of Raab as TP, is obtained. The pre-ejection period includes the time when the electrical impulse is spreading through the ventricle and the time required for tension to build

CHRONODYNOGRAM

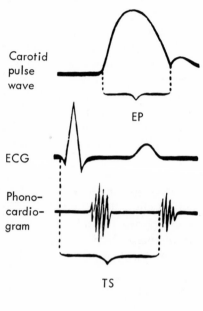

Fig. 12.1 Diagram of the measurement of pre-ejection period (TP) from Raab (294) with permission of the publisher.

TS

TP=TS-EP

up in the ventricle before blood is ejected. At one time this period was erroneously referred to as the isometric period.

The method illustrated in Figure 12.1 was first described by Edens in 1929(33) and later used by Blumberger (33, 34) in Germany and Raab (294) in the United States. In one report (236), changes in PEP in dogs over a wide range as measured by catheter tip micromanometers in the left ventricle and aorta were faithfully reflected in changes in PEP as measured externally by Blumberger method ($r = 0.944$). More recently this was found to be true only at a lower level of end diastolic pressure below 12 mm Hg (349). Left ventricular ejection time as measured externally from the carotid artery has been found to agree with ejection time measured directly in the aorta during cardiac catheterization in humans (19, 369).

There is abundant evidence that a marked augmentation in circulating catecholamines increases rate of tension development in the myocardium which, in turn, is reflected in a shortened PEP (145, 156, 293, 294, 295, 297, 349). Raab concluded, therefore, that resting PEP reflects chronic catecholamine influences on the myocardium and thus its oxygen utilization/supply ratio and perhaps susceptibility to infarction.

Raab (292) has maintained that the critical factor in the state of health of the myocardium is the ratio of oxygen demand to oxgen supply. He has stated that insufficient attention has been paid to oxyged demand, that is, the numerator of the ratio. The study of atherosclerosis, lipid deposition, cholesterol concentration, etc., has to do with oxgen supply, whereas stress is mostly concerned with oxgen demand. In stressful situations, catecholamine production increases, cardiac oxgen demand increases, the coronary arteries dilate, and blood flow is greatly augmented, resulting in 100 percent adaptation. However, Raab postulated if, because of coronary atherosclerosis, the coronary blood flow cannot be increased sufficiently in the face of a stress-related increase in oxygen demand, the cells most distant from the capillaries may lack oxygen and myocardial infarction may result.

We are all familiar with the characteristic bradycardia (low heart rate) of athletes reflecting vagus (i.e., parasympathetic) stimulation. This is sometimes called cholinergic (from acetycholine) dominance as contrasted with adrenergic (from adrenaline) or sympathetic dominace. Raab (292, 294) has presented data to indicate that PEP is influenced by physical conditioning and has concluded that physical inactivity and stress might shift the "cholenergic-adrenergic balance" in the myocardium toward an adrenergic preponderance and a shortened pre-ejection period.

Measurements in Tecumseh

Because the noninvasive method employed by Raab was painless and required relatively little time, it was a feasible one to employ in the large-scale epidemiologic study in Tecumseh. The second series of examinations in this population has thus provided data that bear on Raab's hypotheses.

Approximately 83 percent of the total population of Tecumseh and the rural fringe participated in the second round of clinic examinations in the Tecumseh study. However, with a clinic load of 20 to 35 subjects per day, it was not feasible to determine the pre-ejection period in the entire population. Equipment was available to test only one subject as a time, so measurements could be made on only about 10 percent of the participating subjects. The 646 subjects actually measured did not represent a randomly selected sample of the study population. If the testing station were available, the next available subject, age 10 years or over, was tested. However, if several subjects were available, preference was given to males above age 30. Within any age group, the sample was likely to be representative. However, the total sample is not representative of the community because a higher percentage of older subjects were given the test. In the group of subjects tested, there were 28 men and 16 women who had cardiovascular disease.

The subjects rested quietly for 20 to 30 minutes in a fairly well-lighted, temperature-controlled room (22 to 24° C.) in an attempt to establish a near basal state. A small crystal microphone was placed in a position giving the loudest second heart sound. In many of our subjects the transducer for the arterial pulse was placed over the carotid artery. It was sometimes difficult and time-consuming for a technician to determine the optimum location and pressure for this pulse transducer. A simpler method was sought. By using an infant-size blood pressure bladder in a special long narrow cuff around the subject's neck, with the bladder positioned over the left carotid artery and inflated to a pressure of 10 mm Hg, satisfactory records were obtained regularly. In most cases, using this technique, a prominent wave of the superimposed jugular venous pulse appeared on the finished record but did not interfere with definition of the carotid pressure pulse (259). An eight-channel Electronics for Medicine DR-8 photographic recorder was used with a paper speed of 100 mm/sec and independent time lines at intervals of 0.02 sec.

If the onset of QRS is ascertained from only a single limb or chest lead, it is conceivable that in some instances ventricular depolarization may initially be isolectric in that lead. This could result in an error in which the QS_2 time is underestimated. To ensure that this would not happen, three mutually orthogonal electrocardiograms were recorded with the indirect carotid pulse and phonocardiogram. Figure 12.2 shows a typical recording from one subject. Measurements were made from the first deflection of QRS in any of the three leads. In 97.5 percent of the cases, the Z-lead (chest to back) used alone showed the same time of onset of QRS as when all three leads were used.

The relationship of blood pressure and heart rate to PEP, LVET, and QS_2 was investigated by regression analysis (257). The results indicated it was necessary to correct QS_2, LVET, and PEP for heart rate but not for blood pressure. The resulting normalized values, corrected for heart rate are called QS_2-score, LVET-score, and PEP-score, respectively. The value of 10 was added to eliminate negative scores; hence, when both male and female scores are included, the means of these scores are 10 and the standard deviations are 1.0. Details of the procedure are described elsewhere (257).

Age and Sex Comparisons

For purposes of this analysis, the 44 subjects with cardiovascular disease were excluded. The results on the 602 remaining subjects are presented in Figures 12.3, 12.4, and 12.5. Figures 12.3 and 12.4 show means plus and minus two standard errors of the means for heart rate, QS_2, LVET, and PEP, all uncorrected for heart rate. Figure 12.5 contains these same descriptive statistics for the corrected values.

Normal Values

Our average values for LVET of about 300 msec for males and about 305 msec for females (Figure 12.3) agree very well with what others have reported (19, 33, 136, 154, 157, 222, 233, 367, 368, 373). In one report

PAPER SPEED: 100 mm./sec.   TIME LINES: 0.02 sec.

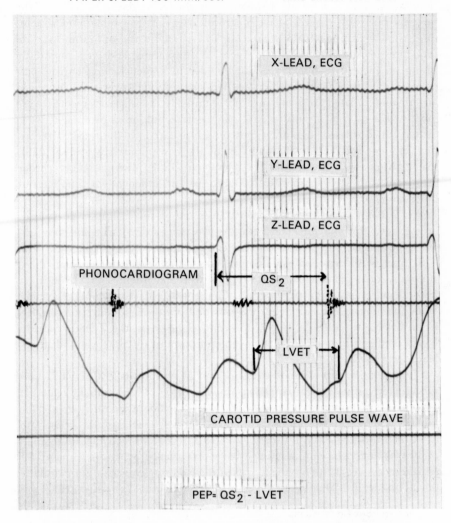

Fig. 12.2 Recording of orthogonal ECG, phonocardiogram, and indirect arterial carotid pulse tracing. Abbreviations: QS_2 (Q-wave of ECG to second heart sound); LVET (Left Ventricular Ejection Time); PEP (Pre-ejection Period). Reproduced from (259) with permission of the publisher.

on infants and young children (156), the values are lower, but this no doubt is due to the high heart rates in young children.

Comparison of our PEP values with other data is more difficult because of possible variations in measurement techniques. In a review by Raab (294) of eight studies in which the measurement was made in much the same way as in the present study, mean values ranged from 82 to 93 msec

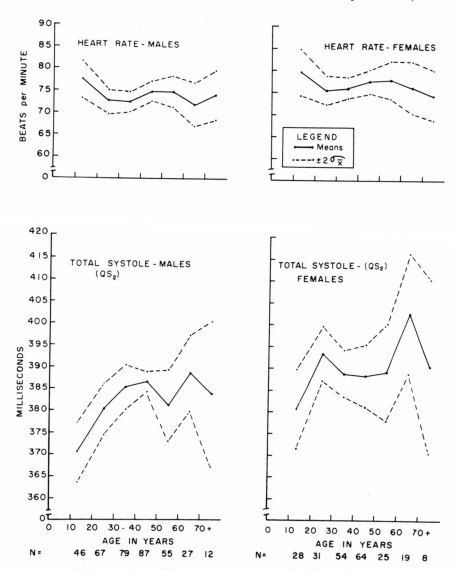

Fig. 12.3 Heart rates (upper graphs) and total systole (lower graphs) for males and females by age group. Reproduced from (257) with permission of the publisher.

in untrained and 85 to 114 msec in trained subjects. Most of these persons were young or middle-aged men. Our mean values for men in these age groups ranged from 80 to 86 msec. Because our respondents for the most part are untrained, the values compare reasonably well with those reported by Raab (294), Blumberger and Sigisbert (33), Frank and Kinlaw (133), Naughton and others (271), and Whitsett and Naughton (373), but slightly

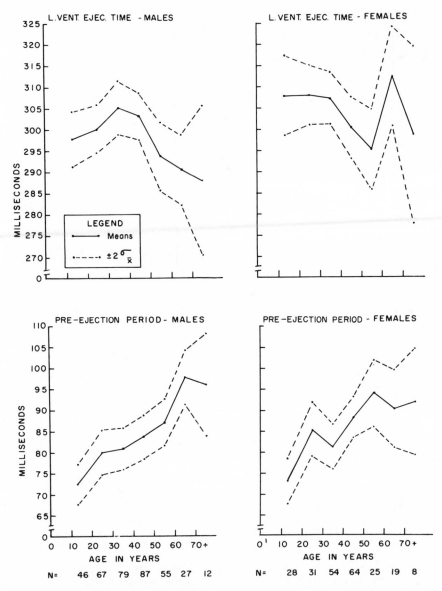

Fig. 12.4 Left ventricular ejection period (upper graphs) and pre-ejection period (lower graphs) for males and females by age group. Reproduced from (257) with permission of the publisher.

lower than those reported by Weissler et al. (367), Molnar et al. (260), and Wiley (375). Metzger, Kroetz, and Leonard (236) reported an average value of 87 msec in dogs. Some investigators measured PEP as the time from

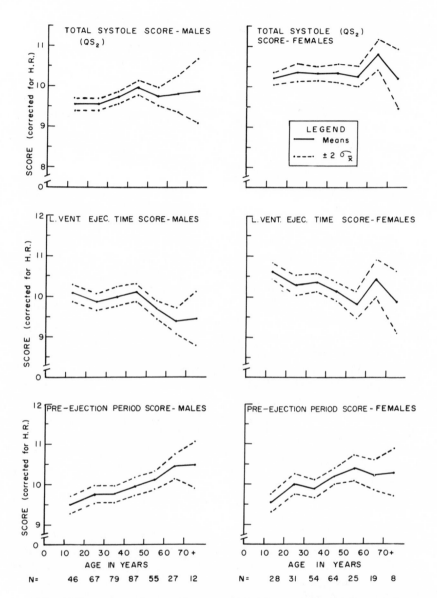

Fig. 12.5 Total systole score (upper graphs), left ventricular ejection period score (center graphs), and pre-ejection period score (lower graphs) for males and females by age group. Reproduced from (257) with permission of the publisher.

the start of QRS of the ECG to the beginning of the indirect carotid pulse wave. These mean values, 127 msec (347), 139 msec (206), 111 msec (377), and 208 msec (124) are greater because they include the transmission time of the pulse wave from the left ventricle to the carotid or radial artery.

Age Differences

Pre-ejection period increased with age in both sexes (Figure 12.4). When corrected for heart rate, the age effect persisted (Figure 12.5). This, in general, agrees with other studies (156, 157, 294). LVET was essentially independent of age, so as PEP increases with age, QS_2 also increases slightly, similar to results of Molnar et al. (260). Harrison et al. (157) and Gobbato and Media (136) reported a slight increase in LVET with age that disappeared when LVET was corrected for heart rate. Lombard and Cope (222) reported no change in total systole with age. Harris et al. (156) measured cardiac isovolumetric time (essentially PEP minus the time from the onset of QRS to the first high-frequency component of the first heart sound) and found this to be shorter in young children. They attributed the results to an increase in the rate of pressure rise in the left ventricle and to a lower diastolic blood pressure in young children. They concluded that the shorter isovolumetric period in children is probably due to greater sympathetic tone (hence an increase in rate of pressure rise) or to a change in the geometry of the heart. Albert, Gale, and Taylor (2) reported that ATPase activity of fresh myofibrils decreased with age. The velocity of shortening and rate of development of isometric force also decrease with age. In our data, because PEP was not related to blood pressure, the increase in PEP with age cannot be attributed to any increase in blood pressure. In all probability, the increase in PEP reflects decreased contractility, supporting the conclusion of Starr: "When one considers the evidence concerning the effect of aging . . . the conclusion is irresistible that the strength of the heart declines as age advances. The heart also tends to lose the fine coordination of its contraction as age advances." (343)

Sex Differences

The higher reclining heart rate in females (Figure 12.3) is well known (11, 235, 256). Left ventricular ejection period, and hence also time of total systole, was greater in females (Figures 12.3 and 12.4), supporting the observations of Lombard and Cope (222) and Weissler and colleagues (367). This is somewhat surprising in view of the lower stroke volume in women (10) and the positive correlation between stroke volume and LVET (40, 136, 368). In our data there was no sex difference in PEP, which is in agreement with observations of Weissler et al. (367). McLean, Clason, and Stoughton (233) also reported no sex difference when PEP was measured from the onset of QRS to the beginning of the rapid ascent of the left ventricular pressure pulse during cardiac catheterization.

Patients with Heart Disease

Data for the 44 patients with cardiovascular disease are compared with normals in Figure 12.6 (PEP) and Figure 12.7 (PEP-Score). Clearly these patients did not have shorter PEP values, as one might expect from

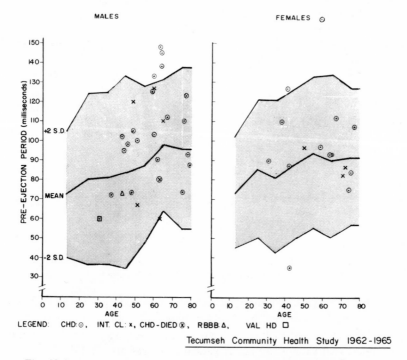

Fig. 12.6 Pre-ejection period; patients with cardiovascular disease compared to normal subjects. Reproduced from (258) with permission of the publisher.

Raab's hypothesis. In fact, PEP tends to be prolonged and LVET to be shortened in these patients (258), to some extent resembling the older heart. Others have recently reported similar results (234, 373, 374). There were no differences in QS_2, corrected or uncorrected for heart rate, between patients and normals (258).

In patients with heart failure, Weissler and colleagues (366–369) reported an increase in PEP which was correlated with a decrease in stroke index. The increase in PEP was balanced by a decrease in LVET so that the duration of electromechanical QS_2 was not different from that in normal subjects.

In Tecumseh patients, as indicated above, there was a prolongation of PEP, because five subjects with coronary heart disease and one with intermittent claudication exceeded the mean of the normal subjects by more than two standard deviations. This might indicate a trend toward decreased

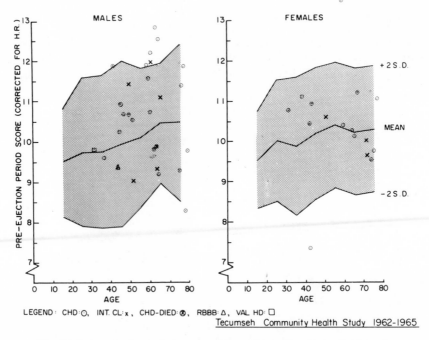

Fig. 12.7 Pre-ejection period score; patients with cardiovascular disease compared to normal subjects. Reproduced from (258) with permission of the publisher.

myocardial contractility in these subjects, as suggested by Weissler and others (366–369), and confirmed by McConahay and colleagues (234). In the latter study, prolonged PEP was shown to be related to a lower stroke volume index, decreased rate of rise of left ventricular pressure, and decreased ejection fraction. A number of animal studies (3, 24, 78, 284, 324) produced convincing evidence for improved contractility as a result of exercise training.

Some of our subjects, knowing of their coronary heart disease, might have altered their habits and outlook on life so as to reduce the stress to which they were subjected. However, it seems more likely that if stress is a causal factor in coronary heart disease or an acute cardiac episode, it is not reflected in the PEP.

Pre-ejection Period and Habitual Physical Activity

As described in Chapter 3, habitual physical activity data were available on 1,129 males, age 16 to 69. The following physical activity indices were used in relating PEP to habitual physical activity.

1. The average number of hours per week of occupational work including all occupations of the respondent.
2. A weighted mean WMR/BMR utilizing the WMR/BMR associated with each of the subject's occupational activities, weighted by the

number of hours spent at each. This reflects the rate of energy expended on the job.
3. Active leisure index, the sum of products for each active leisure pursuit (WMR/BMR × hours spent). This reflects the total energy expenditure during active leisure.
4. A weighted mean WMR/BMR as in number 2 including both occupational and leisure activities. This index reflects the average 24-hour daily rate of energy expenditure.

For the present analysis, data from the following subjects were excluded: (a) men over age 64 because there were too few subjects, (b) those employed less than 10 hours per week at the time of the interview, and (c) those men for whom no information was available on occupation.

Table 12.1 contains a comparison of PEP and PEP-score, among the most active, intermediately active, and least active men. The data were

Table 12.1

HABITUAL PHYSICAL ACTIVITY AND LEFT VENTRICULAR PRE-EJECTION PERIOD AND PRE-EJECTION SCORE

Physical Activity Score	Activity Groups Compared	N	Mean PEP (Milliseconds)	Mean PEP Score
Mean WMR/BMR Occupation and Leisure	Highest	54	78.3	9.70
	Intermediate	148	85.6	9.99
	Lowest	42	82.1	9.87
Mean WMR/BMR Occupation Only	Highest	87	82.9	9.89
	Intermediate	113	83.8	9.93
	Lowest	44	83.1	9.87
Hours Worked per week in Occupation	Highest	39	81.9	9.83
	Intermediate	69	80.2	9.78
	Lowest	136	85.4	9.99
Active Leisure Index	Highest	52	84.9	9.94
	Intermediate	141	82.9	9.89
	Lowest	51	83.0	9.90
Farmers		42	86.9	10.05

analyzed by a one-way analysis of variance comparing mean PEP of each of the three activity groups. This was done in the age-specific groups and then combined over all ages. The analysis was repeated for each of the four physical activity classifications. Data on farmers were not included in the statistical analysis because it was not possible to calculate physical activity indices for them. The mean values for the farmers are included for comparison. None of the F-values, either age-specific or over all ages, was statistically significant at a probability of 0.05. There is also no trend for more active men to have either a higher or lower PEP than the less active men. This analysis was repeated for PEP-score and again no significant *F*-values resulted. When QS_2 and LVET, corrected and uncorrected for heart rate, were studied in the same way, there was no relationship to habitual physical activity (259).

While these data were being analyzed, we were able to compare University of Michigan varsity and freshmen swimmers near the peak of their training with untrained college men of about the same age (172). Table 12.2 shows the comparison. Despite clear evidence that the athletes were highly conditioned (lower heart rate response to exercise and higher maximal oxygen uptake), there was no difference in heart rate-corrected PEP.

Table 12.2

COMPARISONS OF TRAINED FRESHMAN AND VARSITY
SWIMMERS WITH UNTRAINED SUBJECTS

Variable	Trained Athletes (N = 15)	Nonathletes (N = 36)	t	P
Post Exercise Heart Rate (Beats/min)	117.2	141.6	5.8	< 0.001
Max. Vo_2* (ml/kg/min)	56.0	46.9	3.4	< 0.01
Adj. QS_2 (msec)	386	385	0.2	> 0.05
Adj. LVET (msec)	297	295	0.6	> 0.05
Adj. PEP (msec)	89	91	0.6	> 0.05

This measurement was taken on subsamples only. N = 5 for athletes, N = 8 for nonathletes.

Raab (294) and Raab and Krzywanek (292; pp. 121–34) refer to eight population studies including two of their own in which the mean PEP was longer in the more active subjects. However, the statistical significance of the differences is not given and apparently the measurements were not corrected for heart rate. Differences in habitual physical activity in our Tecumseh population may not have been sufficient to demonstrate a difference in PEP, or the method of appraising habitual physical activity may not have been sufficiently precise for subtle differences to be detected. As a counter argument to this, it should be mentioned that more active men classified in the same way were leaner and had lower resting blood pressures, serum total cholesterol, and post-exercise heart rates than the less active subjects. Furthermore, Whitsett and Naughton (373) reported no differences in PEP or LVET between active and sedentary healthy subjects and no significant differences between active and sedentary patients. Additionally, Winters and others (376) actually reported shortened QS_2 and PEP in active compared to inactive subjects!

Many of the studies reported by Raab (292, pp. 121–34) involved athletes or men exposed to strenuous training. Our athlete–nonathlete comparison produced no significant differences in PEP (172). Frick and others (134) also reported no significant differences in heart rate-corrected PEP in trained athletes compared to untrained subjects and cross-country runners had about the same values for PEP and LVET as our untrained subjects of comparable age (271). Fardy (124) reported longer PEP in athletes but these values are in no way comparable because they included the pulse wave transmission time to the radial artery and were not corrected for heart rate.

Effects of Physical Conditioning on the Pre-ejection Period

Raab and Krzywanek (292, pp. 121–34) summarize five reports in which training lengthened PEP, but again the statistical significance of these differences is not given and the values were not corrected for heart rate. Howard's study (172) provided an opportunity to study the effects of training on PEP. Pre-ejection period was recorded in 36 nonconditioned male college students and the Harvard Step Test (43) was then administered. The score was the heart rate in beats per minute from 1 to 1 1/2 minutes after the five-minute exercise. Heart rate response to a standard submaximal exercise has frequently been employed as a rough measure of physical fitness, the higher heart rates during recovery reflecting poorer physical fitness.

Twenty of the subjects (Group A) then trained *hard* 45 minutes a day, 5 days per week, for 5 weeks. Sixteen subjects (Group B) served as controls. At the end of this 5-week period, the subjects were retested and the groups reversed, Group B undertaking strenuous training and Group A serving as a control (detraining). An inspection of Figure 12.8 reveals that the conditioning period improved the fitness of the subjects (lower heart rate response to exercise) and this was reversed with detraining. However, there were no significant changes with conditioning in the heart rate-adjusted resting pre-ejection period.

Frick and colleagues (134) also found no effect of training on heart rate-corrected PEP. Wiley (375) and Fardy's studies (123) likewise showed no effect of training on PEP but these reports are difficult to interpret because PEP is not corrected for heart rate and in Fardy's study PEP is measured without taking into consideration the transmission time of the pulse wave from the heart to the carotid artery. In a recent study, training is reported to increase PEP but it is not stated whether or not the values are corrected for heart rate (138).

The slow heart rates, which characterize trained athletes or people engaged in regular physical exercise, would indicate, as Raab (294) suggested, that hearts of these people are under dominant cholinergic influence. However, other evidence that habitual physical activity is related to adrenergic-cholinergic balance in the myocardium is lacking. Furthermore,

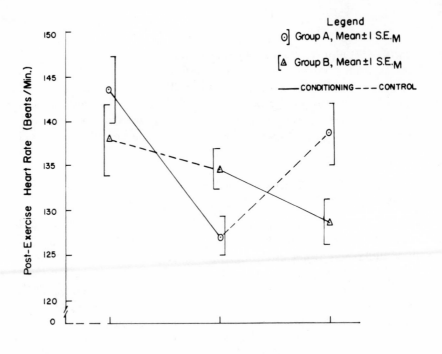

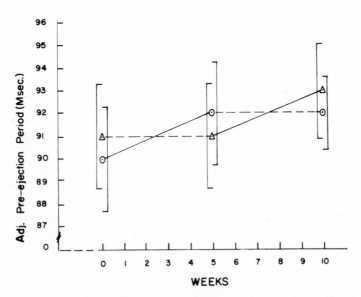

Fig. 12.8 Effects of training (conditioning) on the post-exercise heart rate (upper graph) and the resting or pre-exercise pre-ejection period, adjusted for resting heart rate (lower graph).

the resting stroke volume is larger in athletes and the heart rate is lower, which should lead to greater diastolic stretch. This, in turn might result in the fibers contracting with greater vigor. The rate of pressure increase in the ventricle would be greater, conceivably resulting in a shorter PEP possibly balancing a cholinergic effect. In dogs, shortened time to maximal rate of pressure increase, a measure of contractility, is associated with shortened PEP (349).

Pre-ejection Period and Physical Fitness

All of the subjects in Tecumseh whose resting cardiac pre-ejection period was measured were given a modification of the Harvard Step Test (Chapter 4) unless excluded from the step test for medical reasons. As mentioned above, a higher heart rate following exercise indicates relatively poorer fitness. Correlation coefficients representing the relationship between the one-minute post-exercise heart rates and PEP corrected for heart rate are shown in Table 12.3. There was no significant correlation of post-exercise

Table 12.3

CORRELATION COEFFICIENTS* OF POST-EXERCISE HEART RATE
WITH CARDIAC PRE-EJECTION PERIOD SCORE

Age Group	N	Correlation Coefficient
	Males	
10–19	37	.12
20–29	63	−.15
30–39	72	.05
40–49	66	.00
50–59	33	−.07
60–69	10	.23
	Females	
10–19	24	.09
20–29	29	.11
30–39	49	−.07
40–49	47	−.16
50–59	14	−.46
60–69	5	−.02

*None of these coefficients is statistically significant at $p < .05$.

heart rate with PEP. Our data, showing no correlation of PEP with heart rate response to exercise, support the lack of correlation between PEP and a work capacity test reported by Tharp (359). Tharp reported a significant correlation between QS_2 and work capacity. However, if the influence of heart rate is eliminated in his data by the partial correlation technique, the relationship between QS_2 and work capacity becomes insignificant.

Table 12.4

CORRELATION COEFFICIENTS: LEFT VENTRICULAR PRE-EJECTION PERIOD SCORES WITH STRENGTH AND CERTAIN MORPHOLOGICAL VARIABLES

Age Group	Body Weight		Stature		Sum of Four Skinfolds		Sum of R. & L. Grip Strength		Arm Strength		Cardiac Thoracic Ratio	
	r	N	r	N	r	N	r	N	r	N	r	N
						Males						
10–19	.06	39	−.02	39	.14	39	−.03	38	.00	38	.21	38
20–39	.05	67	.06	67	−.05	67	.13	65	.07	61	−.11	67
30–39	−.06	81	−.19	81	.02	81	−.03	74	−.08	60	.07	81
40–49	.01	94	−.11	94	.09	94	−.18	82	−.17	53	.08	94
50–59	−.18	59	.06	59	−.14	59	−.06	41	.10	26	−.23	59
60–69	.21	34	.09	34	.32	33	−.12	18	.21	9	−.02	34
						Females						
10–19	.17	24	−.24	24	.18	24	.14	23	.00	22	−.07	24
20–29	.12	31	.15	31	.03	31	.19	27	−.14	24	.33	29
30–39	.19	55	−.20	55	.28	55	−.16	49	.02	40	−.07	52
40–49	−.08	66	−.13	67	.03	67	−.05	50	.04	28	.02	64
50–59	.14	28	.29	28	.00	28	.49	20	−.15	10	−.13	27
60–69	.10	22	.21	22	.04	22	.35	10	−.86	3	−.22	22

Table 12.5

CORRELATION COEFFICIENTS: LEFT VENTRICULAR PRE-EJECTION PERIOD SCORES WITH CERTAIN HEMOCHEMICAL AND LUNG FUNCTION MEASUREMENTS

Age Group	Serum Total Cholesterol		Blood Glucose		Serum Uric Acid		Lung Function					
							Vital Capacity		$FEV_{1.0}$		Peak Flow	
	r	N	r	N	r	N	r	N	r	N	r	N
						Males						
10–19	−.23	37	.00	37	.03	30	.00	37	−.07	37	−.06	37
20–29	−.03	67	−.29	67	.07	59	.14	66	.15	66	.28	66
30–39	−.09	80	−.04	79	.04	68	−.01	76	.01	76	.10	76
40–49	.05	94	−.15	94	−.04	90	−.22	82	−.27	82	−.28	82
50–59	.08	58	−.00	59	−.07	54	−.01	55	.00	55	−.13	55
60–69	.06	34	−.12	34	.00	26	.00	27	−.10	27	−.01	27
						Females						
10–19	.16	22	.06	23	.47	16	−.18	23	−.14	23	−.13	23
20–29	.05	31	.11	30	−.20	30	.17	30	.18	30	.00	30
30–39	−.02	55	−.10	55	.17	50	−.11	52	−.22	52	−.12	51
40–49	.07	64	.02	67	−.10	57	−.14	61	−.16	61	−.26	61
50–59	.06	28	−.31	28	−.21	26	.12	24	.17	24	.20	24
60–69	−.10	22	.11	22	−.03	17	.07	18	.06	18	.12	18

Other Relationships

The relationship of PEP, QS_2, and LVET, corrected and uncorrected for heart rate, to body weight, stature, skinfold thickness, arm and grip strength, heart size, serum cholesterol, serum uric acid, glucose tolerance, and pulmonary function (peak flow $FEV_{1.0}$ and vital capacity) were studied. All of the laboratory measurements were taken in the clinic during the same visit, at which the cardiac pre-ejection time was recorded. The methods for blood analyses and pulmonary function are described in previous chapters. The relationships were investigated by calculating correlation coefficients between the cardiac measurements and the other variables within age- and sex-specific groups. There were no statistically significant relationships. The data for PEP-score are summarized in Tables 12.4 and 12.5.

Conclusions

Cardiac pre-ejection period, corrected and uncorrected, for heart rate, increases with age in males and females. There is a tendency for coronary heart disease patients to have a longer PEP, but there is much overlapping with normals. Habitual physical activity and athletic conditioning appeared to be unrelated to PEP in our studies. This is contrary to Raab and Krzywanek (294, pp. 121–34), who reported longer PEP among physically active subjects. However, these investigators did not correct the measurements for heart rate. Also, the classification of their subjects as active or inactive was not explained or supported by other evidence of physical condition. In light of our results and conclusions, the measurement of PEP in the Tecumseh population has been discontinued.

Chapter 13 / Smoking Habits, Chronic Bronchitis, and Lung Function

Smoking habits, chronic bronchitis, and lung function of residents of Tecumseh have been studied by Higgens (Payne) and co-workers (97, 165, 166, 167, 283). With regard to smoking habits, age-sex distributions of nonsmokers, ex-smokers, cigarette smokers, and pipe and cigar smokers have been reported together with the relationship of smoking habits to respiratory symptoms and lung function (283). Cigarette smokers had more respiratory symptoms and, in men, had poorer lung function scores. Familial relationships in smoking habits were found between husbands and wives, between parents and children, and among siblings (167). Cigarette smokers in Tecumseh are also leaner and have lower blood pressures (166) and their parents tended to die at a younger age (97). Proportionally more male cigarette smokers died between the first and second series of examinations in Tecumseh than did nonsmokers (165).

Smoking Habits and Habitual Physical Activity

With regard to the question of whether smoking and occupational physical activity habits are related, conflicting statements have appeared in the literature. Karvonen (193, 195) reported a significantly higher percentage of heavy smokers and lower percentage of nonsmokers among men engaged in a strenuous occupation (lumberjacks) compared to men in other occupations. Similarly, Spain and Nathan (339) found a greater percentage of smokers among heavy workers. In the railroad workers studied by Taylor and his group (205, 352), the percentage of smokers was greater in the more active switchmen. In the study by Stamler and co-workers (23, 340, 341), there appeared to be little or no relation between smoking habits and physical activity of work.

In the investigation by Frank and his associates (132) in which habitual activity was based on occupation and leisure, there was little difference among groups in the percentage of cigarette smokers. When physical activity assessment is based upon leisure only, Lilienfeld (220) and Doan and co-workers (103) found more smokers among the active groups, but Raab and Krzywanek (297) reported slightly more smoking among the less active. Jenkins and others (180) also found more smoking in the least active.

Higgens and collaborators (167) studied smoking habits and occupation in Tecumseh and reported a slight relationship between the two. There was a significantly greater proportion of cigarette smokers, age 20 to 39 and 60 and over, among male blue-collar workers than among other occupational groups. There was little difference in occupation among middle-aged males who smoked cigarettes and those who did not smoke. Among women, relatively more cigarette smokers than nonsmokers held white-collar jobs. However, because occupational classification is not a very precise measure of habitual physical activity, the relationship between smoking habits and habitual physical activity in males as assessed by the methods described in Chapter 3 was studied. Information about smoking habits was obtained by lay interviewers using a standard questionnaire.

When the male subjects (excluding farmers) were classified as smokers or nonsmokers, the percentage of subjects in each category was not much different for the least active, intermediately active, and most active groups. However, in all but one age group there was a smaller percentage of farmers who smoked. An example of these results is shown in Figure 13.1. In this case, the physical activity groups were formed on the basis of an estimate of average 24-hour energy expenditure; i.e., mean WMR/BMR for occupation plus leisure (left side of Figure 13.1) or an estimate of average energy expenditure for active leisure; i.e., leisure index (right side of Figure 13.1). Similarly, there was little correlation between smoking habits and physical activity when subjects were grouped by the other estimates of occupational or leisure activity indices described in Chapter 3. Graphs like Figure 13.1 were also drawn, with cigar and pipe smokers excluded. Because cigar and/or pipe smokers were so few in number, the graphs were almost identical as when the smokers included cigar and pipe smokers. From our results it appears clear that smoking habits among nonfarmers are not responsible for any relationships observed between habitual physical activity and other coronary heart disease risk factors.

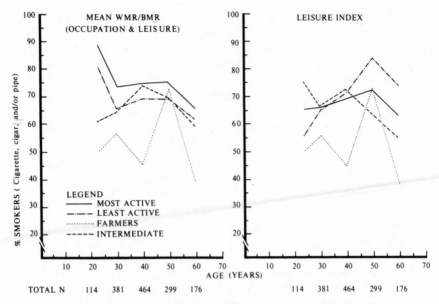

Fig. 13.1 Percentage of males who smoke among physical activity groups based on occupation and leisure (left panel) and leisure activity only (right panel).

Heart Rate Response to Exercise

Smoking Habits

The "chronic" effects of tobacco smoking on the response of man to exercise have not been clearly established. One study reported higher resting heart rates among smokers but no difference in submaximal exercise heart rates (27). In another investigation (58), the heart rates at rest, and three minutes after a standard ride on a bicycle ergometer were significantly higher in smokers. Similarly, submaximal exercise heart rates were higher (hence, predicted maximal oxygen uptake lower) in smokers (286). Giving up smoking decreased the heart rate during and after five minutes (submaximal) exercise (209). Maximal work capacity has long been known to be reduced in smokers (74, 93, 137).

In the present study, respondents were grouped by smoking habits. The numbers in each age group are shown in Table 13.1. An earlier study of the Tecumseh population (166) showed that male and female smokers had significantly higher age-adjusted resting heart rates than nonsmokers. The question then arose: Would heart rates during or after a standard exercise distinguish between the smokers and nonsmokers to a greater extent than the resting rates?

Table 13.1

SMOKING HABITS, LUNG FUNCTION, CHRONIC LUNG DISEASE BY AGE AND SEX, TECUMSEH, MICHIGAN, 1962–1965: NUMBER OF SUBJECTS

	Men Age Groups							Women Age Groups						
	16–19	20–24	25–34	35–44	45–54	55–64	65–69	16–19	20–24	25–34	35–44	45–54	55–64	65–69
	Numbers							Numbers						
FEV$_{1.0}$ Score														
< 8.49	14	19	33	40	19	14	2	16	25	33	19	9	2	—
8.5–8.99	19	16	30	31	21	11	2	10	24	32	31	16	5	—
9.00–10.99	190	141	303	309	161	77	9	176	143	323	331	147	63	—
> 10.99	35	24	61	68	23	13	4	25	16	65	72	32	4	—
Totals	258	200	427	459	235	115	17	227	208	453	453	204	74	—
Smoking Habits														
Nonsmokers	144	48	99	77	38	23	4	197	115	250	246	122	53	3
Cigarette smokers	93	126	250	284	141	56	6	39	94	189	205	69	21	1
Cigar and pipe only	1	12	44	47	28	15	4							
Ex-cigarette smokers	3	12	39	56	25	20	2	4	9	37	35	17	2	—
Totals	241	198	432	464	232	114	16	240	218	476	486	208	76	4
Shortness of Breath														
Moderate and severe	1	3	6	7	6	5	—	6	6	19	23	13	4	—
Mild	7	19	45	48	33	22	1	18	29	68	100	43	17	2
None	247	178	391	414	205	84	16	215	178	383	352	150	54	2
Totals	255	200	442	469	244	111	17	239	213	470	475	206	75	4
Chronic Bronchitis														
Present	7	26	60	84	44	19	4	3	7	20	36	7	4	—
Absent	253	179	383	393	197	97	13	239	210	457	447	203	71	—
Totals	260	205	443	477	241	116	17	241	217	477	483	210	75	—

Reproduced from (86) with permission of the publisher.

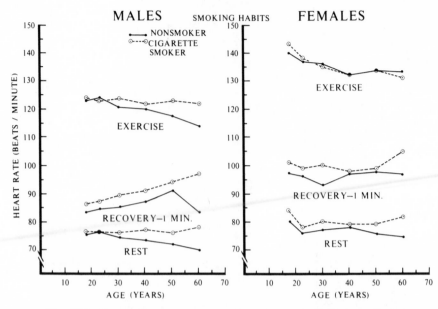

Fig. 13.2 Mean heart rates at rest, exercise, and one minute after exercise for cigarette smokers and for nonsmokers.

The results, reported previously (86), are shown in Figure 13.2. The ex-smokers and cigar and pipe smokers, although included in the statistical analysis, are not represented in Figure 13.2 because the numbers in these groups are small. Their heart rates as a group were higher than nonsmokers but lower than cigarette smokers, on the average. The smokers (i.e., cigarette smokers) in Figure 13.2 have significantly higher exercise and recovery (1 minute post-exercise) heart rates but the differences compared to nonsmokers were about the same as in the case of resting heart rates.

It is also possible that greater differences would have been found if it had been possible to test everyone. Subjects were excluded if they had a history of symptoms of heart disease and chronic respiratory disease, and therefore, more of those not tested were likely to be smokers, especially those more severely affected and less physically fit. Nevertheless, these results are in general agreement with the study by Chevalier and others (58). In studies that showed no difference in exercise heart rates between smokers and non-smokers, the exercise was less vigorous. The higher resting, exercise, and post-exercise heart rates in smokers may reflect greater chronic catecholamine stimulation or possibly some binding of hemoglobin with carbon monoxide. However, it is also possible that the state of fitness is poorer among smokers simply because this group might be less inclined to exercise regularly.

Chronic Bronchitis

Initial information about respiratory illness and symptoms was obtained by lay interviewers. Physicians reviewed this information and supplemented it when the respondents were examined in the clinic. Chronic bronchitis was diagnosed when cough and phlegm were present for at least three months out of the year. Inquiries were made about the presence or absence of shortness of breath which was graded according to severity. Mild shortness of breath was present on walking fast and climbing stairs and when doing strenuous work or exercise; moderate shortness of breath, on walking with other people at ordinary speed; and severe shortness of breath required the subject to stop for breath when walking at his own speed. Not all shortness of breath is due to respiratory disease but no attempt is made here to differentiate between causes of this symptom. The numbers of subjects in each

MALES

ABSENT •——•
PRESENT ⊙----⊙

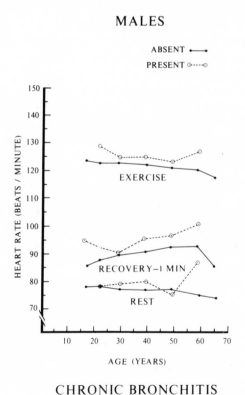

CHRONIC BRONCHITIS

Fig. 13.3 Mean heart rates at rest, exercise, and one minute after exercise for subjects with and without chronic bronchitis.

group are shown in Table 13.1. Subjects with moderate and severe shortness of breath were combined because the numbers were small.

The heart rates for males with and without chronic bronchitis (cough and phlegm) are shown in Figure 13.3. There were few females who reported these symptoms so the results are not shown. Male bronchitics have higher heart rates during and after a standard exercise. The differences compared to nonbronchitics are statistically significant ($p < .05$) over all ages and in several specific age groups. Resting heart rates were also higher in bronchitics but the differences were not as marked.

Table 13.1 also shows the number of subjects in each age-sex group reporting shortness of breath. Figure 13.4 indicates that those respondents who reported shortness of breath have, on the average, higher heart rates before, during, and after exercise. Few male subjects reported moderate or severe shortness; hence, this group was omitted from Figure 13.4.

Although the magnitude of the difference between the heart rates of chronic bronchitics and those subjects without chronic bronchitis is small and often does not reach statistical significance when age-specific comparisons are made, the comparison over all age groups is significant. Apparently, a small but consistent association exists between more favorable heart rate response to exercise and the lack of bronchitic symptoms. Possibly a more strenuous exercise test in which the workload was more precisely controlled, such as a treadmill test, would have shown larger differences be-

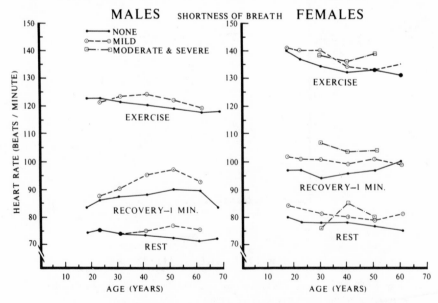

Fig. 13.4 Mean heart rates at rest, exercise, and one minute after exercise for subjects reporting none, mild, moderate and severe shortness of breath.

tween the groups. However, as shown by Jones et al. (182), cardiovascular factors play relatively little part in the limitation of exercise tolerance in patients with chronic airway obstruction. Maximal heart rates for the patients they studied fell short of the maximal value the authors expected for the subjects' ages. Nevertheless, the reduction in exercise tolerance resulting from dyspnea may limit the physical activity of our subjects reporting the presence of cough and phlegm or severe shortness of breath, which in turn would have a detraining effect on the cardiovascular system. In addition, it should be noted that there is considerable overlapping of these subjects with the smokers.

Lung Function

Ventilatory capacity was measured with a Wedge spirometer from which volume and flow were recorded on a Sanborn two-channel recorder. Seven indices were measured from the volume and flow tracings of a maximal forced expiration that followed a maximal inspiration. Two satisfactory tracings were obtained for each subject and measurements were taken from the one with the largest vital capacity. Forced expiratory volume at 1 second ($FEV_{1.0}$) is the volume expired in the first second. In this report, age and height-adjusted $FEV_{1.0}$ Scores were used as the index of ventilatory capacity. The Score was computed as follows: Predicted $FEV_{1.0}$ values were derived for men and women separately from regression equations expressing the relationship of $FEV_{1.0}$ to age and height in persons without cough, phlegm, or shortness of breath. Scores were computed from the formula:

$$FEV_{1.0} \text{ Score} = \frac{\text{Observed } FEV_{1.0} - \text{Predicted } FEV_{1.0} + 10}{\text{standard error of estimate}}$$

The overall mean $FEV_{1.0}$ score for persons without respiratory symptoms is 10; values below this indicate ventilatory lung function below the average for persons of the same sex, age, and height. Subjects were arranged into four groups based upon their $FEV_{1.0}$ scores. The groups consisted of those with scores below 8.50, 8.50 to 8.99, 9.00 to 10.99, and 11.00 and greater. The numbers in each group are given in Table 13.1. These groups overlap with the other categories because many of the same subjects have chronic bronchitis, shortness of breath, low $FEV_{1.0}$ score, and are smokers (283).

Although subjects were classified into four categories on the basis of forced expiratory volume scores, the mean heart rates for only the two groups representing the highest and lowest $FEV_{1.0}$ scores are shown in Figure 13.5. The male subjects who had the highest $FEV_{1.0}$ scores (> 11.00) had lower resting and exercise heart rates. The differences were statistically significant only in the upper age groups. This trend was not as clear in females. In general, lung function as measured by $FEV_{1.0}$ does not appear to be closely correlated with heart rate reponse to submaximal exercise.

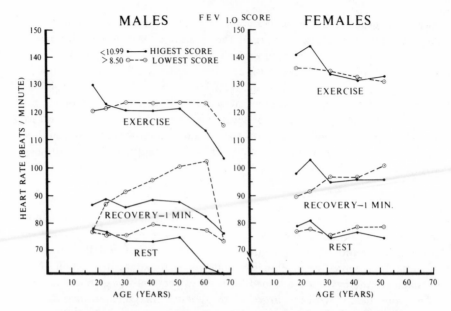

Fig. 13.5 Mean heart rates at rest, exercise, and one minute after exercise for subjects with the highest FEV$_{1.0}$ scores and lowest FEV$_{1.0}$ scores. Intermediate groups were omitted.

Gout

Gout is a disease resulting from a disturbance in protein metabolism. Normally, the end product of purine metabolism in man is uric acid which is excreted by the kidneys (0.5 to 1.0 grams per day). Uric acid is also present in the blood serum—normally 2 to 6 mg percent. In patients with gout, there is either an abnormally high rate of synthesis of uric acid, impairment in its excretion, or both. Generally, in these individuals the concentration of uric acid in the blood and tissues increases, there is deposition of sodium monourate crystals, particularly in cartilage, tendons, and joints, and inflammation results. This is an extremely painful condition. Eventually joint deterioration may result. The disease occurs far more frequently in males than females and rarely occurs in young people. There is evidence of a family history of gout in about 18 percent of the cases (273). Hyperuricemia occurs about five times as often as clinical gout (312).

Measurements in the Tecumseh Study[1]

Serum Uric Acid (SUA) measurements have been made on most of the respondents in Tecumseh, primarily because

[1]The studies reported in this chapter were also supported by the U.S. Public Health Service Research Grant CD00005.

of an interest in the development of arthritis in this population. This has been under the supervision of Dr. W. M. Mikkelsen of the Department of Internal Medicine, Medical Center, University of Michigan and Dr. H. J. Dodge, Department of Epidemiology, School of Public Health, University of Michigan. In the first series of examinations, SUA was determined by the spectrophotometric method of Liddle, Seegmiller, and Laster (219). In the second and third series the autoanalyzer (355) was also used.

Serum Uric Acid, Intelligence, and Achievement

Historians have made the interesting observation that men of genius and distinction are frequently troubled with gout (75, 344). A few examples are Alexander the Great, Francis Bacon, Charlemagne, Lord Chesterfield, Charles Darwin, John Milton, Isaac Newton, and Theodore Roosevelt. This has led one author to speculate that SUA might correlate with intellectual vigor because uric acid shares with certain purines the capacity to stimulate the cerebral cortex (344). It is interesting to note that only in higher apes and man is there a significant amount of uric acid in the blood; lower animals have the capacity to generate hepatic uricase, an enzyme involved in the degradation of uric acid.

Serum Uric Acid in Business Executives

Cobb and his associates (69, 70, 108) have presented evidence that business executives, mostly in the middle management level, had significantly higher levels of SUA than craftsmen. There was a tendency among craftsmen for SUA to be positively related to years of education. It was also reported that medical students, who aspire to a high social level, tended to have high SUA concentrations. Brooks and Mueller (41) reported a positive correlation between SUA values and measures of drive, achievement, and leadership in university professors.

For several years, men in the University of Michigan School of Business Administration Summer Executive Development Program were tested in the Human Performance Laboratory of the University of Michigan. Approximately 90 percent of the executives voluntarily participated in the program. The data on the 167 business executives reported here were collected in the summers of 1962 and 1963. The sample includes 26 bankers, 112 men in executive and middle management positions in public utilities companies, and 29 executives from large corporations throughout the United States. All were between 30 and 50 years of age.

Criteria to clearly define the occupation of an "executive" are difficult to establish. The executives described here varied greatly in their supervisory responsibilities. The group included accountants and legal counsels with limited supervisory responsibilities, as well as general management personnel whose supervisory responsibilities were corporation-wide. All of the men occupied desk positions and were sedentary during most of the working day. This group of business executives provided a unique population that could be compared to the Tecumseh respondents. Dodge and Mikkelsen (105) had previously grouped the men in the Tecumseh population by occupation. The professional men and executives in Tecumseh had higher SUA values than did men in other occupational groups, but the differences were not very striking. The number of managerial positions in a town the size of Tecumseh is, of course, limited.

The serum uric acid determinations for the business executives were done on the autoanalyzer in the same laboratory (William M. Mikkelsen, University of Michigan) by the same technicians during the time when the second-round Tecumseh sera were being analyzed. Only the autoanalyzer values were used in comparing the executives with the Tecumseh population. In a double-blind analysis, repeat determinations were done on sera from a small sample of the executives. There was good agreement. The significantly higher SUA concentration ($p < 0.01$) in the business executives is illustrated in Figure 14.1 confirming the work of Cobb and colleagues (69, 70, 108). Also, Dreyfuss and colleagues (107) showed that SUA is correlated with standard of living in various ethnic groups in Israel.

A much larger percentage of the business executives led sedentary lives (Figure 14.2). However, when matched on the basis of physical activity, the higher SUA in executives persisted (125, 249). These managerial workers also had a higher mean serum total cholesterol level, tended to be fatter, and had higher blood pressure. Correlation of these latter factors with SUA concentration was not sufficiently high to explain the high SUA concentration. Medications taken by the two groups were not studied, but because the men were, for the most part, healthy, this factor was likely important only rarely. It is not clear whether men with high serum uric acid levels are those who tend naturally to be in executive positions or whether the executive's way of life results in an increase in serum uric acid.

Serum Uric Acid and Sports Participation

In view of the thesis by Brooks and Mueller (41) that SUA is positively associated with "drive" and a competitive nature and the reports by Dunn and collaborators (108) and by Kasl and others (198) that high school students who are more active in extracurricular activities have higher SUA, the relationship between sports participation and SUA was studied.

SERUM URIC ACID OF ATHLETES. During the first series of examinations in Tecumseh, it was possible to identify 85 male high school students who

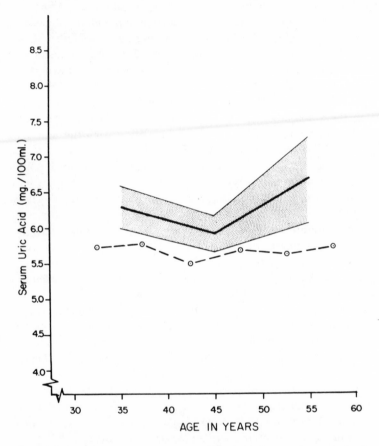

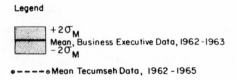

Fig. 14.1 Comparison of business executives with Tecumseh population in serum uric acid concentration. Reproduced from (249) with permission of the publisher.

participated in interschool athletics (253). The age range of the athletes was from 13 to 18 years with a mean of 15.25 years. The distribution of the athletes by sport was as follows: football, 39; baseball, 3; basketball, 5; track, 9; multiple (that is, those who participated in more than one sport), 29. The total males in the Tecumseh population between 13 and 18 years of age included 427 boys. Their mean age was 15.10 years.

PHYSICAL ACTIVITY CLASSIFICATION

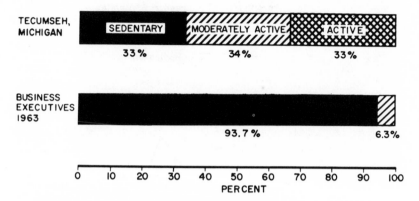

Fig. 14.2 Comparison of business executives and Tecumseh population in habitual physical activity (mean WMR/BMR, occupation and leisure). See Chapter 3 for a description of methods for assessing habitual physical activity. Reproduced from (249) with permission of the publisher.

The SUA concentration was determined by the spectrophotometric method of Liddle, Seegmiller, and Laster (219). The statistical analysis is a little unusual in that the entire Tecumseh male population, age 13 to 18 years of age, was considered the universe of which the athletes constituted a sample. This procedure constitutes sampling from a finite population in which the parameters are known and in which the athlete group constitutes roughly 20 percent of the total population. It was necessary consequently to apply a correction for sampling from a finite population (71).

For age-related measurements such as SUA, the difference between the mean for the athletes and the population mean, at each age, was divided by the standard error of the athlete mean for that age. Under the assumption that the athlete group represents the Tecumseh population, age 13 to 18, t-values were calculated for the various age groups. These may be expected to be approximately normally distributed with a mean of zero and a standard deviation of 6. The sum of the individual t-values across all age levels yielded an age-adjusted t-value for the difference between all athletes and the total population of 2.24, which was statistically significant at $p < .05$. The comparison is shown in Figure 14.3. It should be noted that the subjects in this study were almost all football players who were also fatter (skinfolds) than the age-matched controls (253). Weight and relative weight has been reported to be associated with SUA (264).

Dunn and colleagues (108) had previously reported that 50 high school athletes did not have unusual SUA, but 25 students who excelled academically and also participated in athletics had higher SUA. The higher SUA

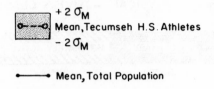

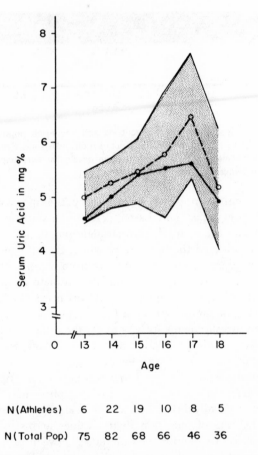

| N(Athletes) | 6 | 22 | 19 | 10 | 8 | 5 |
| N(Total Pop) | 75 | 82 | 68 | 66 | 46 | 36 |

Fig. 14.3 Comparison of athletes with age-matched males in the Tecumseh population in serum uric acid concentration. Reproduced from (253) with permission of the publisher.

in athletes in our report was later confirmed by Greenleaf and colleagues (150) and Thomasson (362), who studied college sportsmen. Horvath (171) reported that international class athletes had higher resting SUA when they were undergoing strenuous athletic training.

Greenleaf and co-workers (150) observed that female physical education instructors, who were likely more active than women of comparable age in the general population, had about the same SUA as other women. Lanese and others (210) also reported no association between SUA and physical activity. Therefore, it seems that those who achieve success in athletics have slightly higher SUA, which is more likely related to personality and motivation to achieve in sports rather than the result of training (chronic exercise). The effect of physical training may be to lower SUA (37, 38, 79, 298) perhaps as a result of expanding the blood volume with training. However, one research group found no change in SUA with physical training (52, 53), so this problem needs further study. The acute effect of exercise is to increase the concentration of SUA (115, 216, 274, 290, 299, 380), probably as a result of decreased urinary flow or a decrease in plasma volume.

SERUM URIC ACID AND ENROLLMENT IN PHYSICAL EDUCATION. SUA was also studied relative to high school electives (Chapter 9). There was no relationship between SUA and the elective high school students selected in Tecumseh (Figure 14.4). None of the F-values applying to Figure 14.4 were significant.

SERUM URIC ACID AND PHYSICAL FITNESS. The physical fitness test scores for children in Tecumseh were compared to their SUA. The age-specific correlation coefficients, with the effects of height, weight, and period between tests removed, are shown in Table 14.1. Only a few coefficients are statistically significant and there is no pattern to these; hence, chance probably is responsible for these significant values.

It is possible that the time lag of from 9 to 38 months between blood sampling and the time when school achievement data were obtained may have vitiated the correlation between the variables. This does not seem likely because SUA is fairly stable over two years ($r = .65$ to $.80$) (198, 264). However, we have no measure of the effect in our data.

Bosco and others (38) also reported no correlation between SUA and step test heart rates, but Allard and Goulet (5) reported a negative relationship between SUA and work performance on a bicycle ergometer in 391 males age 20 to 69. The relationship in the latter study was not a strong one and can be questioned because the effect of age was not controlled.

Serum Uric Acid and Academic Achievement

It was possible to obtain intelligence quotients and educational achievement data on the high school children on whom SUA was available. This is essentially the same sample of the children described in the previous section relating SUA to enrollment in physical education. The numbers at each age, for whom uric acid determinations and other data were available, are shown in Table 14.2. The data on their high school achievement was obtained from the official school records during the 1965 to 1966 school year.

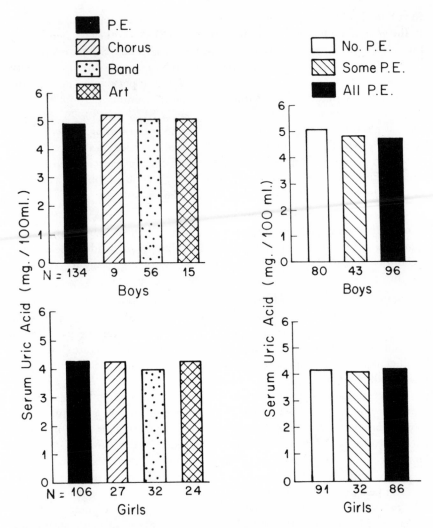

Fig. 14.4 Left side: The relationship of current high school elective and serum uric acid concentration. Mean values are indicated by heights of bars. Right side: Mean serum uric acid of students who elect no physical education, some physical education, or all physical education in high school.

Because the second series of laboratory examinations was conducted from 1961 to 1965, the interval between drawing blood and recording the scholastic data varied from 9 to 38 months. Moreover, serum uric acid increases with age at this time of life, particularly in boys (238). Therefore, a negative correlation between data-collection interval and SUA was anticipated. An analysis of the data confirmed our suspicions. The relationship was found

Table 14.1

CORRELATION COEFFICIENTS: SERUM URIC ACID VS. AAHPER YOUTH FITNESS SCORES
(THE EFFECTS OF HEIGHT, WEIGHT, AND INTERVAL BETWEEN TESTS REMOVED)

Fitness Test	*Age*									
	9	*10*	*11*	*12*	*13*	*14*	*15*	*16*	*17*	*18*
Boys										
Pullups	.07	.07	.31*	.16	.08	-.25*	.29*	.08	.05	-.07
Long Jump	.31	-.09	.16	.24*	.24*	-.24*	.28*	-.01	.12	-.01
Speed in Shuttle Run	.28	.00	.15	.18	.22	-.29*	.01	-.13	.03	.10
Situps	-.25	-.20	.00	.02	.12	-.09	.08	.06	.06	.03
Speed in 50-yd Run	-.09	.27	.13	.14	.30*	-.12	.00	-.18	.27	-.33
Softball Throw	.10	.30*	.00	.19	.21	-.13	.14	-.14	.27	-.23
Speed in 600-yd Run	-.03	-.17	.07	.10	.21	-.26*	.20	-.25	.12	-.12
N=	31	48–49	62	69–73	71–73	65–69	59–65	52–55	53–58	26–28
Girls										
Arm-hang	-.34	-.03	.23	-.13	.02	.11	-.14	-.02	-.04	.39
Long Jump	.10	.03	.33*	.14	.10	-.01	.10	-.36*	.04	.43
Speed in Shuttle Run	.17	.02	.24	.26	.11	-.03	.06	-.40*	-.13	.20
Situps	.00	-.01	.38*	-.29*	.08	.04	-.03	-.10	-.09	.37
Speed in 50-yd Run	-.12	.24	.11	.16	.25	.07	.00	-.20	-.18	-.33
Softball Throw	.03	-.20	.33*	.19	-.09	.19	.16	-.18	.02	.13
Speed in 600-yd Run	-.38*	-.17	.02	.05	-.07	-.04	.03	-.12	-.07	.15
N=	32	48–49	49–53	58	52–56	61–68	65–66	47–54	32–43	10–13

*Statistically significant, p < .05.

Table 14.2

MEANS AND STANDARD DEVIATIONS OF CORRECTED SERUM URIC ACID BY AGE AND SEX

	Boys			Girls		
	Corrected SUA			Corrected SUA		
Age	*Mean*	*SD*	*N*	*Mean*	*SD*	*N*
14*	4.25	1.24	48	4.22	0.90	55
15	4.73	1.17	57	4.23	1.33	62
16	5 03	1.04	52	4.25	0.87	55
17	5.28	1.14	55			⌠39
				4.04	0.90	⎨
18**	5.47	0.90	32			⌊12
Total			244			223

Includes one 13-year-old boy.
**Includes two boys and one girl who were 19 years old.*

to be linear. Regression analysis within each age-sex group was therefore used to correct the SUA for months since clinic visit. The average correction was small, only 0.24 mg percent The means and standard deviations of the corrected SUA are shown in Table 14.2. The corrected SUA values were used in all analyses.

The following data were obtained from the school records:

1. Intelligence quotient: For freshmen, sophomores, and seniors this was calculated from the results of the California Test of Mental Maturity (Short Form, 1963). Juniors had taken the Otis Quick Scoring Test (Gamma Form, E.M.).
2. Academic grade point average (1965–1966 school year).
3. Rank in graduating class (seniors only).

All of the analyses were done separately for boys and girls and by class standing (Freshman, Sophomore, etc.). In all but one set of analyses, the chi square technique was used. It is possible to add the separate chi squares (one for each sex-class standing group) and the degrees of freedom to study the overall relationships. The one exception to using a chi square analysis was in the case of class standing at graduation for seniors. The relationship of class standing and SUA was studied by means of the rank order correlation coefficient (rho).

To illustrate, the relationship between SUA and IQ was studied in freshman boys by tabulating (a) the number of boys in the upper half of the SUA and IQ distributions, (b) those in the upper half of the SUA and lower half of the IQ distributions, (c) those in the lower half of the SUA and upper half of the IQ distributions, and (d) those in the lower half of the SUA and IQ distributions. Under the hypothesis that there is no relationship between

SUA and IQ, one should expect about one-fourth of the subjects in each quadrant. The chi square in this analysis was only 0.01 with one degree of freedom; hence, there is insufficient evidence to reject the hypothesis. Thus one cannot conclude that SUA and IQ are related significantly. The same procedure was followed with the other class standing groups, for boys and girls. The summary of results on the left side of Table 14.3 indicates that SUA and IQ were not related significantly.

Table 14.3

SERUM URIC ACID VS. IQ AND ACADEMIC GRADES

	IQ		Academic Grades	
	Total N	*Chi Square**	*Total N*	*Chi Square**
Boys				
Freshmen	70	0.01	72	2.09
Sophomores	58	0.07	58	1.15
Juniors	48	1.33	47	2.76
Seniors	53	0.92	52	1.58
Total	229	2.33	229	7.58
Girls				
Freshmen	77	0.65	77	0.54
Sophomores	63	1.89	63	1.41
Juniors	34	1.06	34	5.36
Seniors	37	1.33	38	0.22
Total	211	4.93	212	7.53
Grand Total	440	7.26	441	15.11

*None of these chi squares is statistically significant at $p < 0.05$.

Similar analyses were done for the relationship between academic grade point average (1965 to 1966 school year) and SUA. However, each sex-class standing group was divided into approximately three equal subgroups on the basis of academic grades. This provided a series of 2×3 chi square analyses. The results are shown on the right side of Table 14.3. There was no evidence that those children who received high grades had significantly different SUA than those whose grades were low.

Students in the 1966 graduating class were ranked on the basis of their academic grades over the four years in high school. These children were also ranked on the basis of their SUA. As can be seen by the rank order correlations in the first two lines of Table 14.4, there was no significant relationship between SUA and rank in class. Because there is evidence that SUA is related to drive (41), it was thought that perhaps SUA might be higher in "overachievers" in school. Therefore, the seniors were ranked by IQ and academic grades and the difference in these two ranks calculated for each child. Thus, an overachiever would be one whose rank in class was considerably higher than his rank in IQ. These differences in ranks were in turn ranked with highest positive difference (grade rank–IQ rank) at the top. These ranks were then compared with rank in SUA. The coefficients were close to zero (Table 14.4, lines 3 and 4).

Table 14.4

RANK ORDER CORRELATION COEFFICIENTS: SUA RANK
WITH OTHER VARIABLES

Group	Variable	N	Rho*
Senior Males	Rank in Graduating Class	56	0.17
Senior Females	Rank in Graduating Class	40	0.06
Senior Males	Rank of Difference in Ranks	55	0.03
Senior Females	(Graduating Class Rank–IQ Rank)	39	−0.07

*None of these values is statistically significant, $p < .05$

As another way of studying the overachievers, the children who were in the lower half of the IQ distribution in each class standing group were studied separately. These children with the lower IQs were tabulated as to whether they were in the upper or lower SUA distributions and the upper or lower grade point distributions. This provided a 2×2 chi square table for each class standing group. The results are summarized in Table 14.5, which indicates that the overachievers were not different in SUA.

Table 14.5

SERUM URIC ACID VS. ACADEMIC GRADES (GROUPS IN LOWEST
HALF OF SEX-GRADE LEVEL IQ DISTRIBUTION ONLY)

Groups	Total N	Chi Square*
Senior Males and Females	44	1.09
Junior Males and Females	41	2.44
Sophomore Males and Females	58	0.37
Freshman Males and Females	73	0.04
Total	216	3.94

*None of these chi squares is statistically significant, $p < .05$.

The lack of relationship between IQ and SUA is not surprising. Although one investigator (345) reported a statistically significant correlation between these two variables among 817 army recruits, the relationship was very weak ($r = 0.076$). Kasl and collaborators (196, 197) also found a low correlation between IQ and SUA ($r = .10$). Dunn (108) reported no correlation between SUA and college aptitude scores among 96 medical students. Similarly, these investigators reported SUA to be unrelated to grades (high school and medical students) or the difference in grades and aptitude (medical students).

Our results were much the same. On the other hand, Kasl and others (197) reported a significant correlation coefficient ($r = .20$) between SUA and grade point average in high school students. Furthermore, when IQ and grade point average were compared, the overachievers (higher grade point average than would be predicted by their IQ) had significantly higher SUA than underachievers. These results are different from ours. However, Kasl and his group (198) themselves reported varying results in different high schools and postulated that the school setting and selection of subjects may be factors of importance.

Chapter 15 / Relationship of Osteoporosis in Later Life to Habitual Physical Activity

Introduction

According to Garn (139, p. vii), "Bone loss is unquestionably the most common disability of later life. It carries with it the increasing probability of bone fracture. As we now know, bone loss respects neither sex nor race nor geographical area." It is also not partial to long (tubular) bones, round bones, triangular bones, or weight-supporting bones.

Bone is laid down throughout life at the subperiosteal surface (outside surface of the bone) perhaps subject to growth hormone. On the other hand, on the endosteal surface (next to the bone marrow) bone is first lost, then from puberty to about age 30 or 40, bone is added to this inner surface. From about age 40, resorption takes place again. Figure 15.1 illustrates the bone diameters in a typical tubular bone, the second metacarpal.[1] The inner diameter, called the medullary width (M), is bone marrow. The outer diameter is referred to as the total width (T). Subtracting the medullary width from the total width gives the cortical width, or the thickness of the solid bone.

Table 15.1, containing data from the state of Ohio, illustrates that cortical width reaches a maximum at about age 30 to 40 in men and women. Bone loss in later life is about 50 percent greater in women. It has been postulated that this bone loss is just a reflection of muscle loss beyond age 40, but the problem is more complicated than that.

[1]From meta meaning "next to" and carpal for "wrist." The second metacarpal is thus the bone connecting the wrist and index finger.

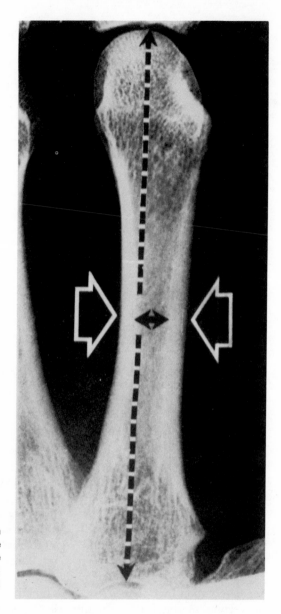

Fig. 15.1 Radiograph of a second metacarpal showing the three measurements taken in the present study. From Garn (140) with permission of the author and publisher.

The likelihood of bone fracture is linearly related to the amount of mineral or bone volume lost (159). It is not surprising, therefore, in view of the data in Table 15.1, that hip fractures increase with age in most populations. In Hong Kong, for example, the incidence in males is 4 per 100,000 at age 40 to 44 and increases steadily to 156 per 100,000 at age 70 to 74. For females the corresponding figures are 2 per 100,000 and 139 per 100,000 (57).

Table 15.1

CHANGING CORTICAL WIDTH IN OHIO WHITES*

Age	Males (mm)		Females (mm)	
	Mean	SD	Mean	SD
1	1.47	0.30	1.49	0.31
2	1.86	0.39	1.81	0.37
4	2.48	0.37	2.34	0.35
6	2.98	0.45	2.78	0.43
8	3.42	0.47	3.22	0.41
10	3.88	0.50	3.54	0.48
12	4.31	0.62	4.16	0.55
14	4.90	0.70	4.87	0.56
16	5.29	0.52	5.08	0.61
18	5.72	0.68	5.16	0.70
22	5.80	0.61	5.31	0.75
30	5.87	0.63	5.36	0.77
40	5.76	0.71	5.46	0.74
50	5.71	0.69	5.23	0.74
60	5.28	0.58	4.56	0.58
70	5.02	0.67	3.99	0.63
80	4.89	0.56	3.30	0.51

*From Garn (*139*, p. 45).
Reproduced from (139), Garn, *The Earlier Gain and Later Loss of Cortical Bone,* with permission of the author and of Charles C Thomas, publisher.

Bone Loss and Physical Activity

For over a century, muscular activity has been known to be essential in the maintenance of normal skeletal volume (159). In the excellent review by Hattner and McMillan (159), three possible mechanisms whereby muscular activity preserves bone integrity are explored. These include (a) direct neural influences on bone, (b) vascular and blood flow changes associated with physical activity, and (c) mechanical stress and strain as a result of weight-bearing and muscular tensions. The third hypothesis best explains the existing data, in the opinion of the authors. Particularly interesting is the observation that bone crystals can function as piezoelectric transducers, converting mechanical strain into electric signals which, in turn, could stimulate bone formation.

When the limbs of monkeys were immobilized, bone resorption took place (223). If a limb is put in a cast, there is a negative calcium balance indicating bone resorption. Several studies of young men in body casts resulted in a loss of about one percent of body calcium in four to six weeks (159). The same results occur in bed rest (159, 178, 223). Astronauts during prolonged space flight experience bone demineralization if they do not exercise. The early Gemini flights produced reductions in radiographic bone density, particularly in the fingers and wrist (159, 223). Weightlessness results in total body calcium loss of about 1 to 2 percent per month. In the Gemini VII flight, exercise appeared to reduce demineralization. Exercise during bed rest has the same effect (223). In certain pathological conditions such as hydrocephalus, in which there is weakness in the limbs because of degeneration or poor development of the pyramidal tracts, the cortical area is reduced. The dynamic nature of bone may be seen in the reduction of cortical area in the femur less than a year after amputation of the lower leg (139, p. 54). Bone loss follows denervation of extremities in cats, rabbits, dogs, and rats (159). However, these are extreme examples of immobility. The question to which we addressed ourselves was, "Are the usual differences in habitual physical activity among men associated with differences in bone loss after age 40?" The Tecumseh Community Health Study provided an opportunity to collect data that bear upon this question (135).

Data from the Tecumseh Community Health Study

Procedures

The data being presented were collected during the second series of examinations in Tecumseh. There was a total of 346 males, aged 45 to 54, for whom a physical activity index (Chapter 3) was available. The men were ranked from the most active to least active. The 50 most active and 50 least active subjects were selected for study. Of these, 3 of the most active and 5 of the least active men did not have hand and wrist X-rays and hence were excluded. A similar procedure was followed in the next age group. Among the 226 men, aged 55 to 64, who had physical activity indices, the 50 most active and least active subjects were selected. Again, because of missing X-rays, there were only 47 men in each group available for study.

Standard anthropometric measurements were taken including stature, weight, arm circumference, and triceps skinfold thickness. Weight was recorded to the nearest kilogram. Standing height, or stature, was recorded to the nearest centimeter. Upper arm circumference in centimeters was measured with a flexible tape midway between the acromion and olecranon processes with the arm hanging freely. Skinfold thickness in millimeters at the triceps was measured with a Lang skinfold caliper having a pressure of approximately 10 grams per square millimeter of contact surface area. The area of muscle and bone at the upper arm (hereafter called muscle area) was computed from the upper arm circumference and triceps skinfold thickness according to Brozek (48). Heart rate response to exercise (see Chapter 4) was available on many of the subjects.

Measurements of cortical bone were derived from micrometric caliper measurements of a 36-inch tube-to-film distance standardized hand-wrist radiographs. Using the dial-reading *Helios* caliper, micrometric measurements were made at the midshaft of the second metacarpal. As illustrated in Figure 15.2, the total subperiosteal diameter (T), the medullary cavity

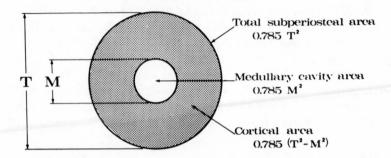

Fig. 15.2 Representations of total subperiosteal area, medullary area, and cortical area as derived from T and M. From Garn (139, p. 11) with permission of the author and publisher.

diameter (M), and length were recorded directly. From this information, assuming the model for a circular tubular bone, the corresponding areas of metacarpal II were calculated as follows:

$$\text{Total Area (mm}^2) = 0.7854 \times T^2$$
$$\text{Medullary Area (mm}^2) = 0.7845 \times M^2$$
$$\text{Cortical Area (mm}^2) = \text{Total Area} - \text{Medullary Area}$$
$$\text{Percent Cortical Area (\%)} = \frac{\text{Cortical Area}}{\text{Total Area}} \times 100$$
$$\text{Cortical Volume (mm}^3) = \text{Length} \times \text{Cortical Area}$$

The widths and areas are correlated with muscle mass because large people tend to have large bones. However, percent cortical area is not related to size, per se, so this measurement is most useful.

These measurements of cortical bone were done under the supervision of A. Roberto Frisancho and Stanley Garn at the Center for Human Growth and Development, University of Michigan. Neither the classification (active or inactive) nor the age of the subject was known to the technician making the X-ray measurements.

Results

The means and standard deviations of all the variables for both age groups are given in Table 15.2. Two-way analyses of variance were performed on all of the variables with the two age groups as one classification

Table 15.2

COMPARISON OF MORPHOLOGICAL VARIABLES OF
SELECTED ADULT MALES OF TECUMSEH, MICHIGAN,
BY AGE AND PHYSICAL ACTIVITY STATUS

	Least Active			*Most Active*		
	N	*Mean*	*SD*	*N*	*Mean*	*SD*
			Age Group: 45–54 Years			
Stature (cm)	45	171.6	5.7	47	173.5	6.4
Weight (kg)	45	77.2	13.1	46	79.0	13.0
Skinfold (mm)	45	15.4	7.2	47	13.9	5.3
Arm Circumference (cm)	45	29.4	3.2	47	29.7	2.7
Arm Muscle Area (cm²)	45	48.6	8.2	47	51.7	9.2
Metacarpal II						
Total Area (mm²)	45	69.9	12.9	47	73.0	10.9
Medullary Area (mm²)	44	11.1	6.6	46	9.4	4.5
Cortical Area (mm²)	44	58.4	9.7	46	62.9	8.2
Percent Cortical Area (%)	44	84.6	7.6	46	87.2	5.1
Cortical Volume (mm³)	44	4051.2	766.3	46	4459.9	724.6
Length (mm)	45	69.3	3.8	47	70.7	4.0
			Age Group: 55–64 Years			
Stature (cm)	47	172.8	6.4	47	170.4	6.1
Weight (kg)	47	76.5	11.4	47	77.1	12.5
Skinfold (mm)	47	16.3	7.4	47	15.2	6.3
Arm Circumference (cm)	47	28.6	2 7	47	29.2	2.9
Arm Muscle Area (cm²)	47	44.1	8.3	47	47.6	7.1
Metacarpal II						
Total Area (mm²)	47	73.6	10.8	47	69.3	10.8
Medullary Area (mm²)	45	12.7	6.6	45	11.7	5.1
Cortical Area (mm²)	45	60.5	8.6	45	57.1	8.0
Percent Cortical Area (%)	45	83.0	7.5	45	83.3	5.7
Cortical Volume (mm³)	45	4223.9	711.1	45	3946.6	684.6
Length (mm)	47	69.8	4.2	47	69.1	4.1

Reproduced from (135) with permission of the publisher.

and the two physical activity groups as the second classification. These analyses indicated that percent cortical area decreased significantly ($p < .05$) and medullary area increased significantly with age. The differences in the activity groups were not significant. However, there were a number of significant interactions including that for the analysis of stature. The least active younger men were shorter, whereas the least active older men were taller. Because taller individuals tend to lose less bone (141), the significant interaction of activity and age with respect to stature could lead to erroneous conclusions. Additional analyses were carried out.

    Analysis of covariance was performed on all the variables with age and stature as covariates. The resulting adjusted mean values and *F*-ratios are given in Table 15.3. These data show that the most active group has a significantly greater area of muscle at the upper arm than the least active group ($p < .01$). The same analyses were carried out with age and arm girth as the

Table 15.3

COMPARISON OF MORPHOLOGICAL VARIABLES ADJUSTED FOR AGE
AND STATURE OF SELECTED ADULT MALES OF TECUMSEH,
MICHIGAN, BY PHYSICAL ACTIVITY STATUS

	Least Active		*Most Active*		
	N	*Mean**	*N*	*Mean**	*F*
Weight (kg)	92	76.8	93	78.1	0.63
Skinfolds (mm)	92	15.8	94	14.5	1.77
Arm Circumference (cm)	92	29.0	94	29.4	1.12
Arm Muscle Area (cm^2)	92	46.4	94	49.6	7.31**
Total Area (mm^2)	92	71.7	94	71.3	0.07
Medullary Area (mm^2)	89	11.9	91	10.6	2.10
Cortical Area (mm^2)	89	59.4	91	60.1	0.25
Percent Cortical Area	89	83.9	91	85.2	1.75
Cortical Volume (mm^3)	89	4132.5	94	4211.9	0.66
Length (mm)	92	69.5	94	80.0	1.05

All mean values were adjusted for age and stature through covariance analyses.
***p < .01.*
Reproduced from (135) with permission of the publisher.

covariates. The resulting F-values are not shown but the only significant ones were for skinfolds and muscle mass. Active males had smaller triceps skinfolds and larger muscle mass when adjusted for age and arm girth.

Comparison of age slopes in the two activity groups demonstrated statistically significant differences only for cortical volume and stature. The difference in slope for stature, of course, was taken into account in the analyses of covariance. As shown in Table 15.4 by the coefficients of correlation and regression, the decrease in cortical bone and arm muscle with the increase in age is comparable in both the most active and least active groups.

Table 15.5 contains zero order correlation coefficients representing the

Table 15.4

CORRELATION OF AGE AND PERCENT CORTICAL AREA AND ARM
MUSCLE AREA FOR SELECTED ADULT MALES OF
TECUMSEH, MICHIGAN

				Regression Equation	
Age Related to:	*N*	*Activity Level*	*r*	*a*	*b*
Percent Cortical Area	91	Most Active	−0.26*	98.68	−0.25X
	89	Least Active	−0.17	95.75	−0.22X
Arm Muscle	94	Most Active	−0.26*	69.57	−0.37X
	92	Least Active	−0.26*	67.52	−0.39X

**p < .05.*
Reproduced from (135) with permission of the publisher.

Table 15.5

CORRELATION MATRIX: PERCENT CORTICAL AREA, AND OTHER VARIABLES OF INTEREST (N IN PARENTHESES)

	Percent Cortical Area	Stature	Weight	Arm Strength	Sum of Right & Left Grip Strengths	Exercise Heart Rate at 2 min 30 sec	Post-Exercise Heart Rate (1 min after ex.)	Right Arm Muscle Area
Age	-.21**(180)	-.10(186)	-.10(185)	-.28*(72)	-.27**(122)	-.01(90)	.16(85)	-.26**(186)
Percent Cortical Area		.01(180)	.01(179)	.10(71)	.12(119)	-.24*(87)	-.28**(81)	.16*(180)
Stature	.01(180)		.44**(185)	.27*(72)	.40**(122)	-.15(90)	-.10(85)	.19**(186)
Weight	.01(179)	.44**(185)		.55**(71)	.41**(121)	.00(89)	.06(84)	.51**(185)
Arm Strength	.10(71)	.27*(72)	.55**(71)		.64**(72)	-.03(52)	-.15(54)	.48**(72)
Sum of Right and Left Grip Strengths	.12(119)	.40**(122)	.41**(121)	.64**(72)		-.23*(76)	-.17(79)	.42**(122)
Exercise Heart Rate at 2 min 30 sec	-.24*(87)	-.15(90)	.00(89)	-.03(52)	-.23*(76)		.72**(79)	-.17*(90)
Post-Exercise Heart Rate 1 min after ex.	-.28**(81)	-.10(85)	.06(84)	-.15(54)	-.17(79)	.72**(79)		.25**(186)
Right Arm Muscle Area	.16*(180)	.19**(186)	.51**(185)	.48**(72)	.42**(122)	-.17(90)	.25**(186)	

*Statistically significant, p < 0.05.
**Statistically significant, p < 0.01.

159

relationships between percent cortical area and other variables of interest. The significant negative correlation with heart rate in the step test suggests that the more fit individuals (lower heart rates) have less bone loss.

Discussion

The findings in this study are both expected and unexpected. They are expected in that they confirm earlier evidence of a reduction with age of bone density, muscle area and muscle strength (139–141). They are unexpected in that the reduction of cortical bone and muscle size with age in the most active group is comparable to that in the least active group. The results, except for the correlations with heart rate response to exercise, do not support the hypothesis of Chalmers (57). He compared various populations (races) and could not explain differences in incidence of bone fracture (senile osteoporosis) by dietary intake of calcium, or hormonal state. Age, which was an important variable, also did not account for the variations among populations, but the incidence in bone fracture did appear to be directly related to standard of living and degree of sedentary living.

These indications would suggest that the effects of activity are noticeable only at the extremes of inactivity or complete immobilization but not at moderate levels. Thus, it is quite possible that only a minimal level of daily physical activity is necessary to maintain a "normal" amount of cortical bone. In support of this argument are the studies that show that even an oscillating bed or quiet standing prevent the negative calcium balance resulting from bed rest. Conversely, it is possible that highter levels of physical activity than the ones considered in the present study may result in a lower rate of bone loss with aging. It is also possible that if the active subjects had been selected on the basis of hand or arm activity only, significant differences may have resulted. This question is being studied with Tecumseh data at the present time.

Buskirk and others (51) made an interesting comparison of the dominant with the nondominant forearm in 7 nationally ranked tennis players. A similar comparison was made in 11 soldiers. A number of significant differences were reported between the two forearms, but there was no significant differences in cortical thickness or diameter of medullary area. Similarly, Sosna (338), in comparing right and left hands of twelve top-ranked fencers, found no differences in bone density despite marked differences in soft tissue. On the other hand, Nilsson and Westlin (275) were able to show significant increases in bone density of the distal end of the femur in 64 young male athletes compared to 39 healthy age-matched nonathletes. Furthermore, among the nonathletes, individuals who exercised regularly had significantly higher density than those who did not. Within the athletes, activities that produced a heavy load on the lower limbs were associated with higher bone density and the leg of preference had a denser femur. A photon-absorption method was used in this study.

It is possible that the method of Nilsson and Westlin is more sensitive and accurate than the X-ray measurement method. This led us to compare the X-ray measurements on most of our subjects with measurements made on the same X-rays by another technician. The correlation coefficients were all .9 or higher.

Serum Total Cholesterol

In all three series of examinations in Tecumseh, blood samples were taken in the clinic. The respondents were not necessarily in a post-absorptive state. Under the supervision of Dr. Walter Block, University of Michigan Medical Center, serum total cholesterol was determined by the Abell (1) or automated method (13).

Relationship to Habitual Physical Activity

Preliminary analyses of the relationship of serum cholesterol with habitual physical activity have been reported (242, 244). More active males were shown to have significantly lower serum total cholesterol than sedentary men. However, the possibility exists that body fatness or perhaps other confounding variables are responsible for the relationships. These analyses are currently being done. Business executives who were more sedentary and fatter than age-matched males in Tecumseh were found to have higher concentrations of serum total cholesterol (125, 248).

Relationship to Enrollment in Physical Education

Enrollment in physical education in high school was determined at the time physical fitness tests were administered to children in Tecumseh as described in Chapter 9. Because serum total cholesterol had been determined 9 to 47 months earlier, the cholesterol values were adjusted for age and for time between assessment of high school elective and cholesterol determination. The adjusted means for boys and girls enrolled in physical education, band, chorus, or art are shown on the left side of Figure 16.1. (See Chapter 9 for details in classification.) Analyses of covariance revealed no statistically significant differences ($p < .05$) in the four groups for either boys or girls.

On the right side of Figure 16.1 is shown a comparison of children who elected physical education all semesters, some semesters, or never elected

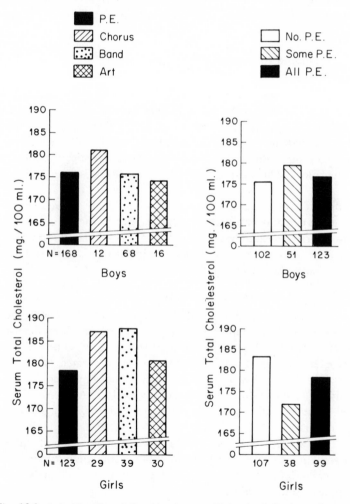

Fig. 16.1 Left side : The relationship of current high school elective and serum total cholesterol concentration. Mean values are indicated by heights of bars. Right side : Mean serum total cholesterol concentration of students who elect no physical education, some physical education, or all physical education in high school.

physical education in high school. Again analysis of covariance revealed no statistically significant difference ($p < .05$) in these adjusted means.

Relationship to Physical Fitness Scores

Age- and sex-specific correlation coefficients for the fitness test scores and serum total cholesterol are shown in Table 16.1. The effects of interval between measurements, height, and weight were removed by partial correlation. There are a few scattered coefficients, significant at a probability of .05, but there is no pattern to these. Hence, they are likely due to chance.

Glucose Tolerance

The correlation of glucose intolerance to diabetes is well-known, but there is evidence that this measurement may also be related to coronary heart disease. When subjects came to the clinic they were given a 50-gram or 100-gram challenge. One hour later, blood was drawn and glucose determined according to the method of Somagyi (337) under the supervision of Dr. Walter Block. The one-hour glucose tolerance test is described by Hayner (162).

A preliminary analysis indicated no significant correlation between glucose tolerance and habitual physical activity as measured in the second Tecumseh series of examinations (242, 244). However, the possible effects of other factors on this relationship are being studied, so these preliminary reports are not to be considered final.

Relationship to Enrollment in Physical Education

The elective that children selected in high school was determined as described in Chapter 9. Glucose tolerance had been determined in most of these children 9 to 47 months earlier during the course of the second series of examinations. The glucose values were corrected for this time lag and age. The adjusted means for the high school boys and girls, grouped by electives, are shown in the left side of Figure 16.2. Analyses of covariance revealed no statistically significant differences ($p < .05$) in the four groups for boys or girls.

On the right side of Figure 16.2 is shown a comparison of children who always, sometimes, or never enrolled in physical education. Again, there were no statistically significant F-values ($p < .05$) as a result of analysis of covariance applied to these adjusted means.

Relationship to Physical Fitness Scores

As for serum cholesterol, age- and sex-specific coefficients of correlation between glucose tolerance values and fitness test scores were

Table 16.1

CORRELATION COEFFICIENTS: SERUM TOTAL CHOLESTEROL VS. AAHPER YOUTH FITNESS SCORES
(THE EFFECTS OF HEIGHT, WEIGHT, AND INTERVAL BETWEEN MEASUREMENTS REMOVED)

Fitness Test	9	10	11	12	13	14	15	16	17	18
					Age					
Boys										
Pullups	-.07	-.08	.12	-.05	-.20	.04	-.16	.05	-.19	-.08
Long Jump	.30	-.17	.29*	.21*	-.17	-.16	-.16	.08	-.16	-.17
Speed in Shuttle Run	.01	-.21	.12	.14	-.14	-.06	-.24*	.14	-.11	-.24
Situps	.04	-.03	.09	.06	.01	-.02	-.06	.10	-.02	.06
Speed in 50-yd Run	.15	.14	.12	.08	-.12	-.15	-.33*	.17	-.04	.13
Softball Throw	.14	-.04	-.14	.23*	.00	-.05	-.24*	.27*	.05	.10
Speed in 600-yd Run	-.24	-.14	.21	.12	-.15	-.03	-.36*	.25*	-.06	.21
N =	39	70–71	85–87	95–99	85–88	83–87	76–83	69–74	66–72	31–34
Girls										
Arm-hang	-.01	-.26*	.01	.13	.19	.08	.12	.08	-.27	-.36
Long Jump	.08	-.05	.15	.22	.17	.00	.13	.23	-.10	-.34
Speed in Shuttle Run	.05	-.12	.23*	.20	.08	.06	.05	.15	-.15	-.53
Situps	.24	-.06	.19	.11	.23	-.06	-.12	.17	.06	-.45
Speed in 50-yd Run	.11	-.16	.20	.14	.13	-.02	-.02	.24	-.26	-.56
Softball Throw	-.02	-.27	.18	.04	-.06	-.20	.10	.22	-.33	-.14
Speed in 600-yd Run	-.14	-.10	.08	-.06	.07	.01	.14	.11	-.20	-.37
N =	45	66–67	69–74	75	63–68	73–80	72–73	54–62	36–51	11–15

Statistically significant, p < .05.

Table 16.2

CORRELATION COEFFICIENTS: BLOOD GLUCOSE VS. AAHPER YOUTH FITNESS SCORES
(THE EFFECTS OF HEIGHT, WEIGHT, AND INTERVAL BETWEEN MEASUREMENTS REMOVED)

Fitness Test	Age									
	9	10	11	12	13	14	15	16	17	18
Boys										
Pullups	.00	-.20	.04	-.19	-.02	-.02	-.12	-.13	.10	.16
Long Jump	.16	-.05	-.21*	-.03	.12	.01	.00	-.07	.06	-.08
Speed in Shuttle Run	-.07	.04	-.23*	-.08	-.07	.12	.00	-.21	-.03	.04
Situps	.15	-.04	-.15	.04	-.13	.21	-.13	-.23	.14	-.03
Speed in 50-yd Run	.21	.05	-.16	-.09	-.03	.16	.12	-.32*	-.03	.14
Softball Throw	.00	.11	-.11	-.01	-.08	.15	.00	-.29*	.10	.15
Speed in 600-yd Run	-.05	.02	-.09	.06	-.05	.18	-.07	-.17	-.20	.13
N =	43	74–75	92–94	97–101	89–91	84–88	80–87	69–73	66–72	31–34
Girls										
Arm-hang	-.06	.10	-.14	.17	-.06	.20	.12	-.09	-.05	.02
Long Jump	.05	.09	.10	-.05	-.10	-.03	-.17	-.15	-.06	.32
Speed in Shuttle Run	.11	.00	.00	-.08	-.10	-.18	-.42*	-.27*	-.17	.05
Situps	-.04	-.01	-.04	-.01	.08	-.05	.13	.07	.29	.36
Speed in 50-yd Run	-.02	.03	.06	.00	-.05	-.09	-.20	-.27*	-.45*	.18
Softball Throw	-.12	.11	-.12	-.08	.04	-.03	-.32*	-.09	-.25	-.19
Speed in 600-yd Run	-.06	.08	.12	-.09	-.04	-.02	-.07	-.12	-.39*	.05
N =	48	67–68	74–79	77	68–73	73–81	71–72	57–66	36–51	12–17

*Statistically significant p < .05.

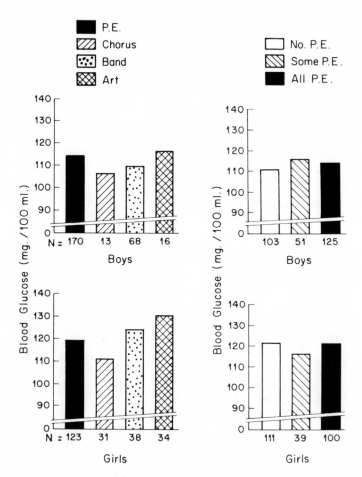

Fig. 16.2 Left side: The relationship of current high school elective and blood glucose one hour after challenge. Mean values are indicated by heights of bars. Right side: Mean blood glucose one hour after challenge of students who elect no physical education, some physical education, or all physical education in high school.

calculated (Table 16.2). The effects of time between measurements, height, and weight were removed by partial correlation. The few scattered statistically significant correlation coefficients were likely due to chance.

Cardiac Diameter

The diameters of the heart and thorax were measured from a standard chest X-ray. The heart diameter was divided by the thoracic diameter to form the cardiac-thoracic ratio.

Relationship to Enrollment in Physical Education

As with serum cholesterol, cardiac thoracic ratios had been calculated for the children in Tecumseh 9 to 47 months before the data on high school enrollment were tabulated. It was necessary therefore to correct the ratios by regression analysis for age and the time interval between measurements. The adjusted means for the physical education, band, chorus, and art groups are compared in the left side of Figure 16.3. As a result of the

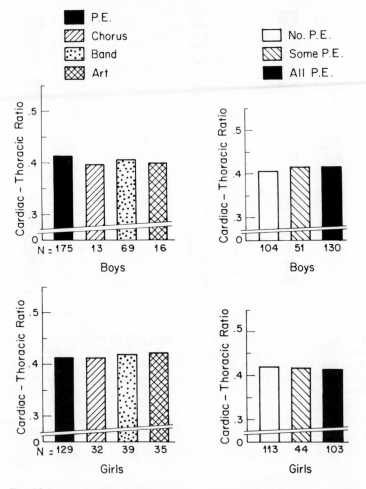

Fig. 16.3 Left side: The relationship of current high school elective and cardiac-thoracic ratio. Mean values are indicated by heights of bars. Right side: Mean cardiac-thoracic ratio of students who elect no physical education, some physical education, or all physical education in high school.

analysis of covariance, neither the F-ratio for the boys or that for girls was statistically significant ($p < .05$).

On the right side of Figure 16.3 is shown the comparison of children who elected physical education all semesters, about half of the semesters, or never elected physical education. Analysis of variance with adjustment for age and time intervals produced an insignificant F-value ($p < .05$) for boys and for girls. These analyses indicate no relation between cardiac-thoracic ratio and enrollment in physical education, on the average, two years later.

Relationship to Physical Fitness Scores

Age- and sex-specific correlation coefficients between the cardiac-thoracic ratios and the fitness test scores, with the effects of time interval, weight, and height removed, are shown in Table 16.3. The few scattered significant ($p < .05$) coefficients are probably due to chance.

Metabolic Capacity and Peridontal Disease[1]

Peridontal disease is a response to an inflammatory process which ultimately results in destruction of the peridontal supporting tissues if it is not arrested. The etiology of the disease is not fully known. Certain factors influence the severity and progression of the disease. Among the most important are age and oral hygiene. However, evidence has been presented implicating other factors including nutrition, occupation, education, income, smoking habits, citric acid metabolism, immune mechanisms, carbohydrate metabolism, personality, and "general resistance to disease." The bone and gingival tissues supporting the teeth are dependent on the circulatory system for nutrients and oxygen. It is possible that individuals who are relatively more fit for strenuous exercise from the standpoint of the cardiovascular-respiratory system (i.e., they have a high maximal oxygen uptake) also may have less peridontal disease. It has also been suggested that persons who are motivated to maintain their general health (proper diet, less smoking, regular exercise) are also those who may practice better oral hygiene. On the other hand, men in the lower socioeconomic levels tend to be the men in occupations involving more physical work. These are the men therefore who might be expected to have a higher oxygen uptake capacity. But lower socio-

[1]The material in this section is described in greater detail in the dissertation by Dr. Richard C. Graves entitled "An Epidemiological Investigation of the Relation between Physiologic Condition and the Severity of Peridontal Disease in Man." The dissertation was submitted in 1971 as partial fulfillment of the requirements for the Doctor of Public Health degree at the University of Michigan.

Table 16-3

CORRELATION COEFFICIENTS: CARDIAC-THORACIC RATIO VS. AAHPER YOUTH FITNESS SCORES (THE EFFECTS OF HEIGHT, WEIGHT, AND INTERVAL BETWEEN MEASUREMENTS REMOVED)

Fitness Test	Age									
	9	10	11	12	13	14	15	16	17	18
Boys										
Pullups	-.05	-.08	.02	.05	-.06	.02	.08	.03	-.19	-.02
Long Jump	-.49*	-.05	.00	-.05	-.23*	-.02	.10	.06	-.02	-.05
Speed in Shuttle Run	-.10	.07	.23*	-.07	-.21	-.18	.12	.15	-.09	-.20
Situps	-.10	-.03	-.02	.20*	-.16	-.05	-.05	.11	-.17	.12
Speed in 50-yd Run	-.33*	-.10	.07	.03	-.13	-.03	.12	.09	-.09	-.10
Softball Throw	-.05	.10	-.03	.07	-.01	.16	.06	.00	-.07	-.16
Speed in 600-yd Run	.27	-.03	-.02	-.18	-.21	.00	.01	.06	.10	-.30
N=	47	88–89	100–102	101–105	88–91	86–91	79–86	72–77	66–72	31–34
Girls										
Arm-Hang	.10	.03	-.14	.07	-.30*	-.12	-.09	-.02	-.30*	.00
Long Jump	.18	.07	.07	-.12	-.10	-.04	-.01	.09	-.07	-.07
Speed in Shuttle Run	.14	.18	.09	-.15	-.22	.08	.08	.11	-.03	-.42
Situps	-.09	.04	-.05	.28*	-.15	-.05	.03	.13	-.09	.06
Speed in 50-yd Run	.08	-.01	.06	-.15	-.29*	-.01	-.02	.11	-.28	.52
Softball Throw	.08	-.08	.02	-.08	-.25*	-.01	.22	.02	-.03	-.02
Speed in 600-yd Run	-.04	.06	-.14	.04	-.06	.07	-.07	.14	-.06	.57
N=	55	80–82	80–85	86	72–77	77–85	74–75	58–67	36–51	14–19

*Statistically significant p < .05.

economic level has also been shown to be related to poorer oral hygiene and hence more peridontal disease.

Among the 543 men, age 35 to 49 years, who were given the treadmill test (Chapter 5) in 1967 to 1969, 486 were available in 1970 to 1971 for a dental examination. Of the 486 men, 64 (13 percent) were edentulous and, hence, excluded from the examination. Of the remaining 422, 34 (8 percent) refused the examination.

Men over age 39 had not exercised to exhaustion. However, from each individual graph of oxygen uptake and heart rate at submaximal workloads, the oxygen uptake at a heart rate of 150 was determined by fitting a straight line by hand. This index ($\dot{V}O_2$ at HR 150) was used as an index of metabolic capacity because the measurement is known to be high in fit, active subjects and low in unfit, sedentary people. The metabolic capacity index was not calculated until after the dental examinations.

The 388 men who were subjects in this study (i.e., those who had had the treadmill test) were all examined by Dr. Graves, who had been a practicing dentist. Four indices were used as follows: (a) Oral Hygiene Index (Green and Vermillion), (b) Decayed, Missing, and Filled Teeth (Korber), (c) Recession Index (Stahl and Morris), and (d) Peridontal Index (Russell).

Metabolic capacity as measured in this study (oxygen uptake at heart rate of 150) was not significantly related to any of the indices of peridontal disease. The level of oral hygiene was also not related to the results of the treadmill test, but less favorable oral hygiene was correlated with greater severity of peridontal disease. The use of tobacco was associated with severity of peridontal disease; however, controlling for oral hygiene status, the relationship was not significant.

References

1. Abell, L. L., B. B. Levy, B. B. Brodic, and F. E. Kendall, "A Simplified Method for the Estimation of Total Cholesterol in Serum and Demonstration of Its Specificity, " *J. Biol. Chem.*, 195, No. 1 (March 1952), 357–66.
2. Albert, N. R., H. H. Gale, and N. Taylor, "The Effect of Age on Contractile Protein ATPase Activity and the Velocity of Shortening," in *Factors Influencing Myocardial Contractility*, R. D. Tanz, F. Kavaler, and J. Roberts, eds. New York: Academic Press, 1967.
3. Aldinger, E. E., "Effects of Digitoxin on the Development of Cardiac Hypertrophy in the Rat Subjected to Chronic Exercise," *Amer. J. Cardiology*, 25, No. 3 (March 1970), 339–43.
4. Alexander, E. R., N. Ting, J. T. Grayston, C. Lu, L. I. Yeou-Bing, and R. A. Bruce, "Pilot Study of Ischemic Heart Disease on Taiwan," *Archives of Environmental Health*, 10, No. 5 (May 1965), 689–93.
5. Allard, C., and C. Goulet, "Physical Working Capacity, Blood Lipids, and Uric Acid," *Sartryck Vr Forsrarsmedicin*, 3, No. 3 (July 1967), 203–205.
6. Anderson, K. L., and A. Elvik, "The Resting Arterial Blood Pressure in Athletes," *Acta Medica Scandinavica*, 153, No. 5 (1956), 367–71.
7. Armstrong, D. B., L. I. Dublin, G. M. Wheatley, and H. H. Marks, "Obesity and Its Relation to Health and Disease," *J. Amer. Med. Assoc.*, 147, No. 11 (November 10, 1951), 1007–1014.
8. Asmussen, E., "Muscular Exercise," *Handbook of Physiology—Respiration II*, pp. 939–978. American Physiology Society, 1965.
9. Åstrand, I., "Aerobic Work Capacity in Men and Women with Special Reference to Age," *Acta Physiologica Scandinavica*, 49, Supplement 169 (February 1960), 1–92.
10. Åstrand, P. O., *Experimental Studies of Physical Working Capacity in Relation to Sex and Age*. Copenhagen: Munksgaard, 1952.
11. ———, "Human Physical Fitness with Special Reference to Sex and Age," *Physiol. Rev.*, 36, No. 3 (July 1956), 307–35.

12. Åstrand, P. O., and B. Saltin, "Oxygen Uptake During the First Minutes of Heavy Exercise," *J. Appl. Physiol.*, 16, No. 6 (November 1961), 971–76.

13. *Autoanalyzer Method for Serum Cholesterol Determination.* Technical Bulletin N24P. Chauncey, N. Y.: Technicon Instruments Corporation, 1963.

14. Baldwin E. de F., A Cournand, and D. W. Richards, Jr., "Pulmonary Insufficiency. I. Methods of Analysis, Physiological Classification, Standard Values in Normal Subjects," *Medicine, Baltimore*, 27, No. 3 (September 1948), 243–78.

15. Baley, J. A., "Recreation and the Aging Process," *Research Quarterly*, 26, No. 1 (March 1955), 1–7.

16. Balke, B., "Correlation of Static and Physical Endurance: I. A Test of Physical Performance Based on the Cardiovascular and Respiratory Response to Gradually Increased Work." Project No. 21-32-004, Report No. 1, U.S.A.F. School of Aviation Medicine, Randolf Field, Texas, April 1952.

17. Balke, B., and R. W. Ware, "An Experimental Study of Physical Fitness of Air Force Personnel," *U.S Armed Forces Medical Journal*, 10, No. 6 (June 1959), 675–88.

18. Bellet, S., M. Eliakim, S. Deliyiannis, and E. M. Figallo, "Radio-electrocardiographic Changes During Strenuous Exercise in Normal Subjects," *Circulation*, 25, No. 4 (April 1962), 686–94.

19. Benchimol, A., E. G. Dimond, and Y. Shen, "Ejection Time in Aortic Stenosis and Mitral Stenosis," *Amer. J. Cardiology*, 5, No. 6 (June 1960), 728–43.

20. Berg, W. E., "Individual Differences in Respiratory Gas Exchange During Recovery from Moderate Exercise," *Amer. J. Physiol*, 149, No. 3 (June 1947), 597–610

21. Berggren, G., and E. H. Christensen, "Heart Rate and Body Temperature as Indices of Metabolic Rate During Work," *Arbeitsphysiologie*, 14 (March 4, 1950), 255–60.

22. Berkson, D. M., J. Stamler, and W. Jackson, "The Precardial Electrocardiogram During and after Strenuous Exercise," *Amer. J. Cardiology*, 18 (July 1966), 43–51.

23. Berkson, D. M., J. Stamler, H. A. Lindberg, W. Miller, H. Mathies, H. Lasky, and Y. Hall, "Socioeconomic Correlates of Atherosclerotic and Hypertensive Heart Disease," *Annals N.Y. Acad. Sci.*, 84 (December 8, 1960), 835–50.

24. Bhan, A. K., and J. Scheuer, "Effect of Physical Conditioning on Cardiac Actomyosin ATPase," *Circulation*, 43–44 Suppl. (October 1971), II–132.

25. Bickelman, A. G., E. J. Lippschutz, and L. Weinstein, "The Responses of Normal and Abnormal Heart to Exercise," *Circulation*, 28, No. 2 (August 1963), 238–49.

26. Blackburn, H., ed., *Measurement in Exercise Electrocardiography.* Springfield, Ill.: Charles C Thomas, 1969.

27. Blackburn, H., J. Brozek, H. L. Taylor, and A. Keys, "Cardiovascular and Related Characteristics in Habitual Smokers and Nonsmokers," Chapter 23 in *Tobacco and Health*, G. James and T. Rosenthal, eds. Springfield, Ill.: Charles C Thomas, 1962, pp. 323–51.

28. Blackburn, H., A. Keys, E. Simonson, P. Rautaharju, and S. Punsar, "The Electrocardiogram in Population Study," *Circulation*, 21, No. 6 (June 1960), 1160–75.

29. Blackburn, H., H. L. Taylor, B. Hamrell, E. Buskirk, W. C. Nicholas, and D.

Thorsen. "The Effect of Physical Conditioning in the Frequency of Ventricular Beats (VPB)," *Circulation*, 46, No. 4 (October 1972), II–12.

30. Blackburn H., H. L. Taylor N. Okamoto, p. Rautaharju, P. L. Mitchell, and A. C. Kerkhof, "Standardization of the Exercise Electrocardiogram. A Systematic Comparison of Chest Lead Configurations Employed for Monitoring During Exercise," in *Physical Activity and the Heart*, M. J. Karvonen and A. J. Barry, eds. Springfield, Ill.: Charles C Thomas, 1967, pp. 101–33.

31. Blackburn, H., H. L. Taylor, C. L. Vasquez, and T. E. Puchner, "The Electrocardiogram During Exercise," *Circulation*, 34, No. 6 (December 1966), 1034–43.

32. Blomqvist, G., "The Frank Lead Exercise Electrocardiogram—A Quantitative Study Based on Averaging Technical and Digital Computer Analysis," *Acta Medica Scandinavica*, 178 (Suppl. 440) (1965), 1–98.

33. Blumberger, K. J., Die Untersuchung der Dynamik des Herzens beim Menschen. Ihre Anwendung als Herzleistungs Prufung. *Ergebnisse der inneren Medizin und Kinderheilkunde*, 62, No. 5 (1942), 424–531.

34. Blumberger, K. J., and M. Sigisbert, "Studies of Cardiac Dynamics," in *Cardiology, an Encyclopedia of the Cardiovascular System*, A. A. Luisada, ed., Vol. 2. New York: McGraw-Hill, 1959, ch. 14: 4–372 to 4–377.

35. *Body Composition in Animals and Man*. Washington, D.C.: Nat. Acad. of Sci., 1968. Publication Number 1598, p. 521.

36. Bookwalter, K. W., "A Study of the Brouha Step Test," *Physical Educator*, 5, No. 3 (May 1948), 55.

37. Bosco, J. S., and J. E. Greenleaf, "Relationships between Hyperuricemia and Gout, Heredity and Behavior Factors, Role of Acute and Chronic Physical Exercise," in *Exercise and Fitness, 1969*, B. D. Franks, ed. Chicago: The Athletic Institute, 1969, pp. 83–95.

38. Bosco, J. S., J. E. Greenleaf, R. L. Kaye, and E. G. Averkin, "Reduction of Serum Uric Acid in Young Men during Physical Training," *Amer. J. Cardiology*, 25, No. 1 (January 1970), 46–52.

39. Božović, L., J. Castenfors, and M. Pescator, "Effect of Prolonged Heavy Exercise on Urine Protein Excretion and Plasma Renin Activity," *Acta Physiologica Scandinavica*, 70, No. 2 (June 1967), 143–46.

40. Braunwald, E., S. J. Sarnoff, and W. N. Stainsby, "Determinants of Duration and Mean Rate of Ventricular Ejection," *Circulation Research*, 6, No. 3 (May 1958), 319–25.

41. Brooks, G.W., and E. Mueller, "Serum Urate Concentrations Among University Professors: Relation to Drive, Achievement and Leadership," *J. Amer. Med. Assn.*, 195, No. 6 (February 9, 1966), 415–18.

42. Brouha, L., *Physiology in Industry*. London: Pergamon Press, 1960, p. 30.

43. ———, "The Step Test: A Simple Method of Measuring Physical Fitness for Muscular Work in Young Men," *Research Quarterly*, 14, No. 1 (March 1943), 31–36.

44. Brown, R., T. McKeown, and A. Whitfield, "Environmental Influences Affecting Arterial Pressure in Males in the Seventh Decade," *Canad. J. Biochem. and Physiol.*, 35, No. 11 (November 1957), 897–911.

45. Brozek, J., "Body Composition," *Science*, 134, No. 3483 (September 29, 1961), 920–30.

46. ———, ed., "Body Composition," Parts I and II, *Annals of N.Y. Acad. Sci.*, 110: 1–1018, 1963.

47. ———, ed., *Body Measurements and Human Nutrition*. Detroit: Wayne State University Press, 1956, p. 167.

48. ———, "Body Measurements Including Skinfold Thickness, as Indicators of Body Composition," in *Techniques for Measuring Body Composition*, J. Brozek and A. Henschel, eds. National Academy of Sciences, National Research Council, Washington, D.C., 1961.

49. Bruce, R. A., and T. R. Hornsten, "Exercise Stress Testing in Evaluation of Patients with Ischemic Heart Disease," Progress in *Cardiovascular Disease*, 11, No. 5 (March 1969), 371–90.

50. Bruce, R. A., and J. R. McDonough, "Stress Testing in Screening for Cardiovascular Disease," *Bull. N.Y. Acad. Med.*, 45, No. 12 (December 1969), 1288–1305.

51. Buskirk, E. R., K. L. Anderson, and J. Brozek, "Unilateral Activity and Bone and Muscular Development in the Forearm," *Research Qtly.*, 27, No. 2 (May 1956), 127–31.

52. Calvy, G. L., L. D. Cady M. A. Mufson et al., "Serum Lipids and Enzymes. Their Levels after High Calorie, High Fat Intake and Vigorous Exercise Regimen in Marine Corps Recruit Personnel," *J. Amer. Med. Assn.*, 183, No. 1 (January 5, 1963), 87–90.

53. Calvy, G. L., L. H. Coffin, M. M. Gertler, and L. D. Cady, "The Effect of Strenuous Exercise on Serum Lipids and Enzymes," *Military Medicine*, 129, No. 11 (November 1964), 1012–16.

54. Castenfors, J., "Renal Function During Exercise," *Acta Physiologica Scandinavica*, 70, No. 3–4 (July–August 1967), 1–44.

55. Castenfors, J., and M. Piscator, "Renal Haemodynamics, Urine Flow and Urinary Protein Excretion during Exercise in Supine Position at Different Loads," *Acta Medica Scandinavica*, Suppl. 472 (1967), pp. 231–44.

56. Cerretelli, P., R. Sikano, and L. E. Farhi, "Readjustments in Cardiac Output and Gas Exchange During Onset of Exercise and Recovery," *J. Appl. Physiol.*, 21, No. 4 (July 1966), 1345–50.

57. Chalmers, J., "Geographical Variations in Senile Osteoporosis: The Association with Physical Activity," *J. Bone and Joint Surgery*, 52, No. 4 (November 1970), 667–75.

58. Chevalier, R. B., J. A. Bowers, S. Bondurant, and J. C. Ross, "Circulatory and Ventilatory Effects of Exercise on Smokers and Non-Smokers," *J. Appl. Physiol.*, 18, No. 2 (March 1963), 357–60.

59. Chiang, B. N., E. R. Alexander, R. A. Bruce, and D. J. Thompson, "Factors Related to ST Segment Depression after Exercise in Middle-Aged Chinese Men," *Circulation*, 40, No. 3 (September 1969), 315–25.

60. Chiang, B. N., E. R. Alexander, R. A. Bruce, and N. Ting, "Physical Characteristics and Exercise Performance of Pedicab and Upper Socio-economic Classes of Middle-Aged Chinese Men," *Amer. Heart Journal*, 76, No. 6 (December 1968), 760–68.

61. Chiang, B. N., H. J. Montoye, and D. A. Cunningham, "Treadmill Exercise Study of Healthy Males in a Total Community—Tecumseh, Michigan: Clini-

cal and Electrocardiographic Characteristics," *Amer. J. Epidemiol.*, 91, No. 4 (April 1970), 368–77.

62. Chiang, B. N., L. V. Perlman, L. D. Ostrander, and F. H. Epstein, "Relationship of Premature Systoles to Coronary Heart Disease and Sudden Death in Tecumseh Epidemiologic Study," *Annals of Internal Medicine*, 70, No. 6 (June 1969), 1159–66.

63. Chiang, B. N., L. V. Perlman, and F. H. Epstein, "Overweight and Hypertension: A Review," *Circulation*, 34, No. 3 (March 1969), 403–21.

64. Chin, A. K., and E. Evanuk, "Changes in Plasma Catecholamine and Corticosterone Levels after Muscular Exercise," *J. Appl. Physiol.*, 30, No. 2 (February 1971), 205–207.

65. Chrastek, J., J. Adamirova, and J. A. Kral, "On the Physical Ability of Juveniles with High Blood Pressure," *Proceedings 15th Internatl. Cong. Sports Med.*, 1964, Tokyo, pp. 58–64.

66. Christensen, E. H., "Beitrage zue Physiologie schwerer korperlicher Arbeit," *Arbeitsphysiologie*, 4, No. 6 (May 1931), 470–502. Quoted by L. Brouha, *Physiology in Industry*. New York: Pergamon Press, 1960, 18.

67. Clarke, A. C., "Use of Leisure and Its Relation to Levels of Occupational Prestige," *Amer. Sociol. Rev.*, 21, No. 3 (June 1956), 301–307.

68. Cobb, L. A., and W. P. Johnson, "Hemodynamic Relationships of Anaerobic Metabolism and Plasma Free Fatty Acids During Prolonged, Strenuous Exercise in Trained and Untrained Subjects," *J. Clinical Investigation*, 42, No. 6 (June 1963), 800–810.

69. Cobb, S., "Hyperuricemia in Executives," in *The Epidemiology of Chronic Rheumatism*, J. H. Kellgren, M. R. Jeffrey, and J. F. A. Ball, eds. Philadelphia: Davis Company, 1963, pp. 182–88.

70. Cobb, S., J. P. Dunn, G. Brooks, G. P. Rodman, "Serum Urate Levels in Males by Social Class," *Arthritis and Rheumatism*, 4 (August 1961), 412.

71. Cochran, W. G., *Sampling Technique*, 2nd ed. New York: John Wiley & Sons, 1963, p. 23.

72. ———, "Some Methods for Strengthening the Common χ^2 Tests," *Biometrics*, 10, No. 4 (December 1954), 417–51.

73. Consolazio, C. F., R. E. Johnson, and L. J. Pecora, *Physiological Measurements of Metabolic Functions in Man*. New York: McGraw-Hill, 1963, 8.

74. Cooper, K. H., G. O. Gey, and R. A. Battenberg, "Effects of Cigarette Smoking on Endurance Performance," *J. Amer. Med. Assn*, 203, No. 3 (January 15, 1968), 189–92.

75. Copeman, W. S. C., *A Short History of Gout and Rheumatic Diseases*. Berkeley and Los Angeles, California: University of California Press, 1964, 236.

76. Cornfield, J., "Joint Dependence of Risk of Coronary Heart Disease in Serum Cholesterol and Systolic Blood Pressure: A Discriminant Function Analysis," *Federation Proceedings*, 21, No. 4, Part II (July–August 1962), 58–61.

77. Costill, D. L., R Bowers, G. Branam, and K. Sparks, "Muscle Glycogen Utilization during Prolonged Exercise on Successive Days," *J. Appl. Physiol.*, 31, No. 6 (December 1971), 834–38.

78. Crews, J., and E. E. Aldinger, "Effect of Chronic Exercise on Myocardial Function," *Amer. Heart Journal*, 74, No. 4 (October 1967), 536–42.

79. Cronau, L. H., Jr., P. J. Rasch, J. W. Hamby, and H. J. Burns, "Effects of Strenuous Physical Training on Serum Uric Acid Levels," *J. Sports Med. and Phys. Fitness*, 12, No. 1 (March 1972), 23–25.

80. Cullumbine, H., "Relationship Between Body Build and Capacity for Exercise," *J. Appl. Physiol.* 10, No. 3 (September 1949), 155–68.

81. ———, "Relationship Between Resting Pulse Rate, Blood Pressure and Physical Fitness," *J. Appl. Physiol.*, 2, No. 5 (November 1941), 278–82.

82. ———, "Survey of Physical Fitness in Ceylon," *Lancet*, 2, No. 6589 (December 1949), 1067–71.

83. Cullumbine, H., S. W. Bibile, T. W. Wikramanayake, and R. S. Watson, "Influence of Age, Sex, Physique and Muscular Development on Physical Fitness," *J. Appl. Physiol.*, 10, No. 9 (March 1949), 488–511.

84. Cumming, G. R., "The Frequency and Possible Significance of Ischemic S-T Changes in the Exercise Electrocardiogram," Chapter 3 in *Training: Scientific Basis and Application*, A. W. Taylor, ed. Springfield, Ill: Charles C Thomas, 1972, 39–59.

85. Cumming, G. R., L. Borysyk, and C. Dufresne, "The Maximal Exercise ECG in Asymptomatic Men," *Canad. Med. Assn. Journal*, 106 (March 18, 1972), 649–53.

86. Cunningham, D. A., H. J. Montoye, M. W. Higgens, and J. B. Keller, "Smoking Habits, Chronic Bronchitis and Shortness of Breath and Physical Fitness," *Medicine and Science in Sports*, 4, No. 3 (Fall 1972), 138–45.

87. Cunningham, D. A., H. J. Montoye, H. L. Metzner, and J. B. Keller, "Active Leisure Activities as Related to Occupation," *J. Leisure Research*, 2, No. 2 (Spring 1970), 104–111.

88. ———, "Active Leisure Time Activities as Related to Age Among Males in a Total Population," *J. Gerontol.*, 23, No. 4 (October 1968), 551–56.

89. ———, "Physical Activity at Work and Active Leisure as Related to Occupation," *Medicine and Science in Sports*, 1, No. 3 (September 1969), 165–70.

90. Cunningham, D. A., H. J. Montoye, and H. G. Welch, "An Evaluation of Equipment for Determining Oxygen Uptake," *Research Qtly.*, 40, No. 4 (December 1969), 851–56.

91. Cureton, T. K., Jr., *Physical Fitness Workbook*, 3rd ed. St. Louis: C. V. Mosby Co., 1947.

92. Dauber, T. R., W. B. Kannel, A. Kagan, R. K. Donabedian, P. McNamara, and G. Pearson, "Enviromental Factors in Hypertension," in *Epidemiology of Hypertension*, J. Stamler, R. Stamler, and T. N. Pullman, eds. New York: Grune and Stratton, Inc., 1967, pp. 255–88.

93. David, K. H., "Age, Cigarette Smoking, and Tests of Physical Fitness," *J. Appl. Psych.*, 52, No. 4 (August 1968), 296–98.

94. Davies, H., N. Gazetopoulas, and C. Oliver, "Ventilatory and Metabolic Response to Graded and Prolonged Exercise in Normal Subjects," *Clin. Sci.*, 24 (December 1965), 443–52.

95. De Schryver, C., P. De Herdt, and J. Lammerant, "Effect of Physical Training on Cardiac Catecholamine Concentrations," *Nature* (London), 214, No. 5091 (May 1967), 907–908.

96. De Schryver, C., J. Mertens-Strythagen, I. Becsei, and J. Lammerant, "Effect of Training on Heart and Skeletal Muscle Catecholamine Concentration in Rats," *Amer. J. Physiol.*, 217, No. 6 (December 1969), 1589–92.

97. Deutscher, S., and M. W. Higgens, "The Relationship of Parental Longevity to Ventilatory Function and Prevalence of Chronic Nonspecific Respiratory Disease among Sons," *Amer. Rev. Respiratory Disease*, 102, No. 2 (August 1970), 180–89.

98. DeVilla, M., V. S. Banka, G. Lee, S. G. Meister, and R. H. Helfant, "Correlation of Quantitative Submaximal Exercise of Ectopia with Coronary Arteriography and Coronary Collaterals," *Circulation*, 46, No. 4 (October 1972), II-145.

99. Dill, D. B., "Assessment of Work Performance," *J. Sports Med. and Phys. Fitness*, 6, No. 1 (March 1966), 3–8.

100. ———, "The Economy of Muscular Exercise," *Physiol. Rev.*, 16, No. 2 (April 1936), 263–91.

101. ———, "A Measure of Health—The Capacity of an Individual for Work," Part II, Section 4 in *Interpretations of Physical Education, Vol. IV, Physiological Health*, Jay B. Nash, ed. New York: A. S. Barnes and Co., 1933, pp. 29–34.

102. Dill, D. B., J. H. Talbott, and H. T. Edwards, "Studies in Muscular Activity. VI. Response to Several Individuals to a Fixed Task," *J. Physiol.*, 69, No. 3 (May 1930), 267–305.

103. Doan, A. E., D. R. Peterson, J. R. Blackmon, and R. A. Bruce, "Myocardial Ischemia after Maximal Exercise in Healthy Men," *Amer. Heart Journal*, 69, No. 1 (January 1965), 11–21.

104. ———, "Myocardial Ischemia after Maximal Exercise in Healthy Men, One Year Follow-Up of Physically Active and Inactive Men," *Amer. J. Cardiol.*, 17, No. 1 (January 1966), 9–19.

105. Dodge, H. J., and W. M. Mikklesen, "Association of Serum Uric Acid Scores with Occupation," *J. Occupational Med.*, 10, No. 8 (August 1968), 402–7.

106. Dowell, L. J., "Recreational Pursuits of Selected Occupational Groups," *Research Qtly.*, 38, No. 4 (December 1967), 719–22.

107. Dreyfuss, F., E. Yaron, and M. Balough, "Blood Uric Acid Levels in Various Ethnic Groups in Israel," *Amer. J. Med. Sci.*, 247, No. 4 (April 1964), 438–44.

108. Dunn, J. P., G. W. Brooks, J. Mausner, G. P. Rodman, S. Cobb, "Social Class Gradient of Serum Uric Acid Levels in Males," *J. Amer. Med. Assn.*, 185, No. 6 (August 10, 1963), 431–36.

109. Durnin, J. V. G. A., and V. Mikulici, "The Influence of Graded Exercise on the Oxygen Consumption, Pulmonary Ventilation and Heart Rate of Young and Elderly Men," *Qtly. J. Experimental Physiol.*, 41, No. 4 (October 1956), 442–52.

110. Edward, R. H. T., D. M. Denison, G. Jones, C. T. M. Davies, and E. J. M. Campbell, "Changes in Mixed Venous Gas Tensions at Start of Exercise in Man," *J. Appl. Physiol.*, 32, No. 2 (February 1972), 165–69.

111. Eklund, L. G., "Circulatory and Respiratory Adaptations During Prolonged Exercise in the Supine Position," *Acta Physiologica Scandinavica*, 68, Nos. 3–4 (November–December 1966), 382–96.

112. ———, "Circulatory and Respiratory Adaptation During Prolonged Exercise of Moderate Intensity in the Sitting Position," *Acta Physiologica Scandinavica*, 69, No. 4 (April 1967), 327–40.

113. Ellestad, M. H., W. Allen, M. C. K. Wan, G. L. Kemp, "Maximal Treadmill Stress Testing for Cardiovascular Evaluation," *Circulation*, 39, No. 4 (April 1969), 517–22.

114. Elliott, D. H., and J. E. Howell, "Causes and Consequences of Differential Leisure Participation among Females in Halifax, Nova Scotia," Chap. 22 in *Training: Scientific Basis and Application,* A. W. Taylor, ed. Springfield, Ill.: Charles C Thomas, 1972, pp. 213–21.

115. Ende, M., "Physiological Effects of Golf," *Virginia Med. Monthly,* 93 (January 1966), 29–32.

116. Epstein, F. H., "An Epidemiological Study in a Total Community: The Tecumseh Project," *U. Mich. Med. Bull.,* 26 (September 1960), 307–314.

117. ———, "The Epidemiology of Coronary Heart Disease: A Review," *J. Chronic Diseases,* 18 (August 1965), 735–74.

118. Epstein, F. H., and R. D. Eckoff, "The Epidemiology of High Blood Pressure— Geographic Distributions and Etiological Factors," in *Epidemiology of Hypertension,* J. Stamler and R. Stamler, eds. New York: Grune and Stratton, Inc., 1967, pp. 155–66.

119. Epstein, F. H., and S. W. Hoobler, "Relationship Between Hypertension and Coronary Atherosclerosis," *Heart Bull.,* 15, No. 6 (November–December 1966), 104–109.

120. Epstein, F. H., et al., "The Tecumseh Study: Design, Progress, and Perspectives," *Archves of Environmental Health,* 21, No. 3 (September 1970), 402–407.

121. Espenschade, A. S., "Restudy of Relationships Between Physical Performance of School Children and Age, Height, and Weight," *Research Qtly.,* 34 (May 1963), 144–53.

122. Evard, E., "Use and Value of the Step Test in Military Pilot Selection," *U.S. Armed Forces Med. Journal,* 10, No. 6 (June 1959), 659–74.

123. Fardy, P. S., "Effects of Soccer Training and Detraining upon Selected Cardiac and Metabolic Measures," *Research Qtly.,* 40, No. 3 (October 1969), 502–508.

124. ———, "The Influence of Physical Activity on Selected Cardiac Cycle Time Components," *J. Sports Med. and Phys. Fitness,* 11, No. 4 (December 1971), 227–33.

125. Faulkner, J. A., H. J. Montoye, and G. W. Greey, "A Comparison of Executives with a Total Population in Physical Activity and Other Possible Coronary Heart Disease Risk Factors," *Med. and Sci. in Sports,* 1, No. 3 (September 1969), 160–64.

126. Faulkner, J. A., D. E. Roberts, R. L. Elk, and J. Conway, "Cardiovascular Responses to Submaximum and Maximum Effort Cycling and Running," *J. Appl. Physiol.,* 30, No. 4 (April 1971), 457–61.

127. Fischer, J. E., W. D. Horst, and I. J. Kopin, "Norepinephrine Metabolism in Hypertrophied Rat Hearts," *Nature* (London), 207, No. 5000 (August 28, 1965), 951–53.

128. Francis, Thomas, Jr., "Aspects of the Tecumseh Study," *Public Health Reports,* 76, No. 11 (November 1961), 963–66.

129. ———, "Biological Aspects of Environment," *Industrial Med. and Surgery,* 30, No. 9 (September 1961), 347–79.

130. ———, "Research in Preventive Medicine," *J. Amer. Med. Assn.,* 172, No. 10 (March 5, 1960), 993–99.

131. Francis, Thomas, Jr., and F. H. Epstein, "Tecumseh, Michigan," *Milbank Memorial Fund Qtly.,* 43, No. 21 (April 1965), 333–42.

132. Frank, C. W., E. Weinblatt, S. Shapiro, and R. V. Sager, "Myocardial Infarc-

tion in Men: Role of Physical Activity and Smoking in Incidence and Mortality," *J. Amer. Med. Assn.*, 198, No. 12 (December 19, 1966), 1241–45.

133. Frank, M. N., and W. B. Kinlaw, "Indirect Measurement of Isovolumetric Contraction Time and Tension Period in Normal Subjects," *Amer. J. Cardiology*, 10, No. 12 (December 1962), 800–806.

134. Frick, M. H., T. Somer, and R. P. Elovainio, "Effect of Physical Training on Left Ventricular Systole," *Cardiologia*, 51, No. 1 (June 1967), 33–45.

135. Frisancho, A. R., H. J. Montoye, M. E. Frantz, H. Metzner, and H. J. Dodge, "A Comparison of Morphological Variables in Adult Males Selected on the Basis of Physical Activity," *Med. and Sci in Sports*, 2, No. 4 (Winter 1970), 209–212.

136. Gabbato, F., and A. Media, "Analysis of the Factors that May Influence the Duration of Isotonic Systole in Normal Conditions," *Cardiologia*, 29, No. 2 (August 1956), 114–31.

137. Galloway, R. W., *Anatomy and Physiology of Physical Training*. London: Bradford and Dickens, 1937, p. 149.

138. Gandee, R. N., J. R. Anthony, R. L. Bartels, R. R. Lanese, and G. L. Fox, "Effect of Interval Training on Systolic Time Intervals," *The Physiologist*, 15, No. 3 (August 1972), 141.

139. Garn, S. M., *The Earlier Gain and Later Loss of Cortical Bone*. Springfield, Ill.: Charles C Thomas, 1970.

140. Garn, S. M., C. G. Rohmann, and P. Nolan, Jr., "The Developmental Nature of Bone Changes during Aging," Chap. 4, in *Relations of Development and Aging*, J. E. Birren, ed. Springfield, Ill.: Charles C Thomas, 1964.

141. Garn, S. M., C. G. Rohmann, and B. Wagner, "Bone Loss as a General Phenomenon in Man," *Federation Proceedings*, 26, No. 6 (November–December 1967), 1729–36.

142. Gauer, O. H., and H. L. Thron, "Postural Changes in the Circulation," Chapter 67 in *Handbook of Physiology Section 2: Circulation*, Vol. III, W. F. Hamilton and P. Dow, eds. Washington, D.C.: The American Physiological Society, 1965.

143. Gilbert, R., J. H. Auchincloss, and G. H. Baule, "Metabolic and Circulatory Adjustments to Unsteady–State Exercise," *J. Appl. Physiol.*, 22, No. 5 (May 1967), 905–912.

144. Goldschlager, N., D. Cake, and K. Cohn, "Significance of Exercise-Induced Ventricular Arrhythmias," *Circulation*, 46, No. 4 (October 1972), II–73.

145. Goldstein, I. M., W. J. De Groat, and J. J. Leonard, "Influence of Exercise and Automatic Tone on the Duration of Left Ventricular Isoventric Contraction," *Circulation*, 24 (October 1961), 942.

146. Gordon, E. S., "Metabolic and Endocrine Factors in Weight Control," Chap. 13, in *Weight Control*. Ames, Ia: Iowa State College Press, 1955.

147. Gore, I. Y., "Physical Activity and Aging—A Survey of Soviet Literature. II. The Effect of Exercise on the Various Systems of the Organism," *Gerontologia Clinica*, 14, No. 2 (1972), 70–77.

148. Grande, F., J. E. Monagle, E. R. Buskirk, and H. L. Taylor, "Body Temperature Responses to Exercise in Man on Restricted Food and Water Intake," *J. Appl. Physiol.*, 14, No. 2 (March 1959), 194–98.

149. Graybeal, L., "Measurement of Outcomes of Physical Education for College Women," *Research Qtly*, 7, No. 4 (December 1936), 60–63.

150. Greenleaf, J. E., R. L. Kaye, and J. S. Bosco, "Elevated Serum Uric Acid Concentration in College Athletes: A Preliminary Study," *Amer. Corrective Therapy Journal*, 23, No. 3 (May/June 1969), 66–69.

151. Grimby, G. N., J. Nilsson, and H. Sanne, "Repeated Serial Determination of Cardiac Output During 30 Minute Exercise," *J. Appl. Physiol.*, 21, No. 6 (November 1966), 1750–56.

152. Gross, E. A., and J. A. Casciani, "The Value of Age, Height and Weight as a Classification Device for Secondary School Students in the Seven AAHPER Youth Fitness Tests," *Research Qtly*, 33, No. 1 (March 1962), 51–58.

153. Guber, S., H. J. Montoye, D. A. Cunningham, and S. Dinka, "Age and Physiological Adjustment to Continuous, Graded Treadmill Exercise," *Research Qtly.*, 43, No. 2 (May 1972), 175–86.

154. Hanson, J. S., B. S. Tabakin, A. M. Levy, and W. Nedde, "Long-Term Physical Training and Cardiovascular Dynamics in Middle-Aged Men," *Circulation*, 38, No. 4 (October 1968), 783–99.

155. Harris, E. A., and B. B. Porter, "On the Heart Rate During Exercise, and Esophageal Temperature and the Oxygen Debt," *Qtly. J. Experimental Physiol.*, 43, No. 3 (July 1958), 313–19.

156. Harris, L. C., A. M. Weissler, A. O. Manske, B. H. Danford, G. D. White, and W. A. Hammill, "The Deviation of the Phases of Mechanical Systole in Infants and Children," *Amer. J. Cardiology*, 14, No. 4 (October 1964), 448–55.

157. Harrison, T. R., K. Dixon, R. O. Russell, P. S. Bidwai, and H. N. Coleman, "The Relation of Age to the Duration of Contraction, Ejection, and Relaxation of the Normal Human Heart, "*Amer. Heart Journal*, 67, No. 2 (February 1964), 189–99.

158. Hathaway, M. L., and E. D. Foard, *Heights and Weights of Adults in the United States*. Washington, D.C.: U.S. Gov't Printing Office, Home Economics Research Report, No. 10, 1960.

159. Hattner, R. S., and D. E. McMillan, "Influence of Weightlessness upon the Skeleton: A Review, "*Aerospace Medicine*, 39, No. 8 (August 1968), 849–55.

160. Haun, Paul, *Recreation: A Medical Viewpoint*. New York: Teachers College, Columbia University, 1965, p. 3.

161. Havighurst, R. J., "The Nature and Values of Meaningful Free-Time Activity," in *Aging and Leisure*, R. W. Kleemier, ed. New York: Oxford University Press, 1961, pp. 309–44.

162. Hayner, N. S., "The One-Hour Oral Glucose Tolerance Test." National Center for Health Statistics. Series 2, Number 3, U.S. Department of Health, Education and Welfare, July 1963.

163. Henschel, A., *Physical Fitness in Old Age*. Occupational Health Program, U.S. Public Health Service. A working paper for the Scientific Group on the Optimal Level of Physical Performance Capacity for Adults, Geneva, Switzerland, October 22–28, 1968. Quoted by E. Simonson, *Physiology of Work Capacity and Fatigue*. Springfield, Ill.: Charles C Thomas, 1972, p. 418.

164. Henschel, A., F. de la Vega, and H. L. Taylor, "Simultaneous Direct and Indirect Blood Pressure Measurements in Man at Rest and Work," *J. Appl. Physiol.*, 6, No. 8 (February 1954), 506–508.

165. Higgins, M. W., and J. B. Keller, "Predictors of Mortality in the Adult Population of Tecumseh," *Archives of Evironmental Health*, 21, No. 3 (September 1970), 418–24.

166. Higgens, M. W., and M. Kjelsberg, "Characteristics of Smokers and Non-Smokers in Tecumseh, Michigan. II. The Distribution of Selected Physical Measurements and Physiologic Variables and the Prevalence of Certain Diseases in Smokers and Non-Smokers," *Amer. J. Epidemiol.*, 86, No. 1 (July 1967), 60–77.

167. Higgens, M. W., M. Kjelsberg, and H. Metzner, "Characteristics of Smokers in Tecumseh, Michigan. I. The Distribution of Smoking Habits in Persons and Families and Their Relationship to Social Characteristics," *Amer. J. Epidemiol.*, 86, No. 1 (July 1967), 45–59.

168. Hill, A. V., and H. Lupton, "Muscular Exercise, Lactic Acid and the Supply and Utilization of Oxygen," *Qtly. J. Med.*, 16 (1923), 135–71.

169. Hodgkins, J., and V. Skubic, "Cardiovascular Efficiency Test Scores for College Women in the United States," *Research Qtly.*, 34, No. 4 (December 1963), 454–61.

170. Holmgren, A., and B. Pernow, "The Reproducibility of Cardiac Output Determination by the Direct Fick Method During Muscular Work," *Scandinavian J. Clin. and Lab. Investigation*, 12, No. 2 (1960), 224–27.

171. Horvath, G., "Blood-Serum Level of Uric Acid in Top Sportsmen," *Acta Rheumatologia Scandinavica*, 13 (1967), 308–312.

172. Howard, G. E., *A Study of the Relationship between the Tension ("Isometric") Period of the Left Ventricle and Physical Training of Young Adult Men.* Ann Arbor, Michigan: Ph. D. Dissertation, University of Michigan, 1968.

173. Howell, W. H., *Textbook of Physiology.* Philadelphia: W. B. Saunders Co., 1930.

174. Humerfelt, S., and F. Wedervang, "A Study of the Influence Upon Blood Pressure of Marital Status, Number of Children and Occupation," *Acta Medica Scandanavica*, 159, No. 6 (1957), 489–97.

175. Hundley, J. M., "Need for Weight Control Programs," Chap. 1, in *Weight Control.* Ames, Ia: Iowa State College Press, 1955.

176. Hunsicker, P. A., and G. C. Reiff, *A Survey and Comparison of Youth Fitness, 1958–1965.* U.S. Office of Education, Report of Cooperative Research, Project No. 2418. Ann Arbor, Mich.: University of Michigan, 1965.

177. Hunter, D., *The Diseases of Occupations.* Boston: Little, Brown and Co., 1962, p. 11.

178. Issekutz, B., J. J. Blizzard, N. C. Birkhead, and K. Rodahl, "Effect of Prolonged Bed Rest on Urinary Calcium Output," *J. Appl. Physiol.*, 21, No. 3 (May 1966), 1013–20.

179. Jelinek, V. M., P. Schweitzer, R. Gorlin, and M. V. Herman, "A Multivariable Exercise Test to Diagnose Coronary Artery Disease," *Circulation*, 46, No. 4 (October 1972), II–73.

180. Jenkins, C. D., S. J. Zyzanski, R. H. Roseman, and M. Friedman, "Epidemiologic Study of Cigarette Smokers and Nonsmokers," *Circulation*, Suppl. III, 40 (November 13–16, 1969), 114.

181. Johnson, B. C., F. H. Epstein, and M. C. Kjelsberg, "Distributions and Family Studies of Blood Pressure and Serum Cholesterol Levels in a Total Community —Tecumseh, Michigan," *J. Chronic Diseases*, 18 (1965), 147–60.

182. Jones, N. L., G. Jones, and R. H. T. Edwards, "Exercise Tolerance in Chronic Airway Obstruction," *Amer. Rev. Respiratory Disease*, 103, No. 4 (April 1971), 479–91.

183. Jones, W. B., R. N. Finchum, R. O. Russell, Jr., and T. J. Reeves, "Transient Cardiac Output Response to Multiple Levels of Supine Exercise," *J. Appl. Physiol.*, 28, No. 2 (February 1970), 183–89.

184. Jones, W. B., and T. J. Reeves, "Total Cardiac Output Response During Four Minutes of Running," *Amer. Heart Journal*, 76, No. 2 (August 1968), 209–16.

185. Jose, A. D., F. Stitt, and D. Collins, "The Effect of Exercise and Changes in Body Temperature on the Intrinsic Heart Rate in Man," *Amer. Heart Journal*, 79, No. 4 (April 1970), 488–98.

186. Kachadorian, W. A., and R. E. Johnson, "The Effect of Exercise on Some Clinical Measures of Renal Function," *Amer. Heart Journal*, 82, No. 2 (August 1971), 278–80.

187. Kaminer, B., and W. P. W. Lutz, "Blood Pressure in Bushmen of the Kalahari Desert," *Circulation*, 22, No. 2 (August 1960), 289–95.

188. Kang, B. S., S. J. Song, C. S. Suh, and S. K. Hong, "Changes in Body Temperature and Basal Metabolic Rate of the Ama," *J. Appl. Physiol.*, 18, No. 3 (May 1963), 483–88.

189. Kapaller-She, A. M., "Prehypertensive State in Residents of Peking," *Klinicheskaya Meditsina*, 40 (1962), 79. Translation in *Federation Proceedings*, 22 (1963), 778–81 (Translation Supplement).

190. Kaplan, M., *Leisure in America*. New York: John Wiley & Son, Inc., 1960.

191. ———, "The Use of Leisure," in *Handbook of Social Gerontology*, C. Tibitts, ed. Chicago: University of Chicago Press, 1960, pp. 407–43.

192. Kaplinsky, E., W. B. Hood, B. McCarthy, L. McCombs, and B. Lown, "Effects of Physical Training in Dogs with Coronary Artery Ligation," *Circulation*, 37, No. 4 (April 1968), 556–65.

193. Karvonen, M. J., "Arteriosclerosis: Clinical Surveys in Finland," *Proceedings*, Royal Society of Medicine, 55 (April 1962), 271–74.

194. ———, "The Relationship of Habitual Physical Activity to Disease in the Cardio-vascular System," in *Physical Activity in Health and Disease*, K. Evang and K. L. Andersen, eds. Baltimore: The Williams and Wilkins Co., 1966, pp. 81–89.

195. Karvonen, M. J., P. M. Rautaharju, E. Orma, S. Punsar, and J. Takkunen, "Cardiovascular Studies on Lumberjacks," *J. Occupational Med.*, 3 (February 1961), 49–53.

196. Kasl, S. V., G. W. Brooks, and S. Cobb, "Serum Urate Concentrations in Male High School Students," *J. Amer. Med. Assn.*, 198 (November 14, 1966), 713–16.

197. Kasl, S. V., G. W. Brooks, and W. L. Rodgers, "Serum Uric Acid and Cholesterol in Achievement Behavior and Motivation. I. The Relationship to Ability, Grades, Test Performance, and Motivation," *J. Amer. Med. Assn.*, 213, No. 7 (August 17, 1970), 1158–64.

198. Kasl, S. V., G. W. Brooks, and W. L. Rodgers, "Serum Uric Acid and Cholesterol in Achievement Behavior and Motivation. II. The Relationship to College Attendance, Extra–curricular and Social Activities, and Vocational Aspirations," *J. Amer. Med. Assn.*, 213, No. 8 (August 24, 1970), 1291–99.

199. Kasser, I. S., and R. A. Bruce, "Comparative Effects of Aging and Coronary Heart Disease in Sub-maximal and Maximal Exercise," *Circulation*, 39, No. 6 (June 1969), 759–74.

200. Kemp, G. L., and M. H. Ellestad, "The Significance of Hyperventilative and Orthostatic T-wave Changes on Electrocardiogram," *Archives of Internal Medicine*, 121, No. 6 (June 1968), 518.

201. Kenyon, G. S., "The Significance of Adult Physical Activity as a Function of Age, Sex, Education, and Socio-Economic Status," Paper presented at the Midwest District Convention of the American Association for Health, Physical Education, and Recreation, Detroit, Michigan, 1964.

202. Keys, A., "Weight Changes and Health of Men," Chap. 8, in *Weight Control*. Ames, Ia.: Iowa State College Press, 1955.

203. Keys, A., and J. Brozek, "Body Fat in Adult Man," *Physiolog. Rev.*, 33, No. 3 (July 1953), 245–325.

204. ———, "Overweight versus Obesity and the Evaluation of Calorie Needs," *Metabolism*, 6, No. 5 (September 1957), 425–34.

205. Keys, A., et al., "Epidemiological Studies Related to Coronary Heart Disease: Characteristics of Men Aged 40–59 in Seven Countries," *Acta Medica Scandanavica Supplement*, 460 (1967), 1–392.

206. Kossman, C. E., and H. H. Goldberg, "Sequence of Ventricular Stimulation and Contraction in a Case of Anomolous Atrioventricular Excitation," *Amer. Heart Journal*, 33, No. 3 (March 1947), 308–18.

207. Kostolna, M., and V. Kirilcukova, "Protein Content after Excretion in Children at Experimental Athletic Schools of the First Degree," *Acta Facultatis Educationis Fisicae Universitatis*, 7 (1968), 95–103.

208. Kraus, H., and W. Raab, *Hypokinetic Disease*. Springfield, Ill.: Charles C Thomas, 1961.

209. Krumholz, R. A., R. B. Chevalier, and J. C. Ross, "Cardiopulmonary Function in Young Smokers: A Comparison of Pulmonary Function Measurement and Some Cardiopulmonary Responses to Exercise Between a Group of Young Smokers and a Comparable Group of Non-Smokers," *Annals Internal Medicine*, 60, No. 4 (August 1964), 603–10.

210. Lanese, R. R., G. E. Greshman, and M. D. Keller, "Behaviorial and Physiological Characteristics in Hyperuricemia," *J. Amer. Med. Assn.*, 207, No. 10 (March 10, 1969), 1878–82.

211. Lapiccirella, V., "Emotion-Induced Cardiac Disturbances and Possible Benefits from Tranquil Living," *Prevention of Ischemic Heart Disease: Principles and Practices*, W. Raab, ed. Springfield, Ill.: Charles C Thomas, 1966, pp. 212–16.

212. Leedy, H. E., A. H. Ismail, W. V. Kessler, and J. E. Christian, "Relationships Between Physical Performance Items and Body Composition," *Research Qtly*, 36, No. 2 (May 1965), 158–63.

213. Leon, A. S., W. D. Horst, and M. A. Saviano, "Effects of Chronic Exercise on Heart Adrenal and Brain Catecholamine Levels," *The Physiologist*, 15, No. 3 (August 1972), 195.

214. Lester, F. M., L. T. Sheffield, and T. J. Reeves, "Electrocardiographic Changes in Clinically Normal Older Men Following Near Maximal and Maximal Exercise," *Circulation*, 36, No. 1 (July 1967), 5–14.

215. Levi, L., "Life Stress and Urinary Excretion of Adrenaline and Noradrenaline,"

in *Prevention of Ischemic Heart Disease: Principles and Practices*, W. Raab, ed. Springfield, Ill.: Charles C Thomas, 1966, pp. 85–95.

216. Levine, S. A., B. Gordon, and C. L. Derick, "Some Changes in the Chemical Constituents of the Blood Following a Marathon Race with Special Reference to the Development of Hypoglycemia," *J. Amer. Med. Assn.*, 82, No. 22 (May 31, 1924), 1778–79.

217. Levy, A. M., B. S. Tabakin, and J. S. Hanson, "Cardiac Output in Normal Men During Steady-State Exercise Utilizing Dye-Dilutional Technique," *British Heart Journal*, 23, No. 4 (July 1961), 425–32.

218. Lewis, H. E., J. Mayer, and A. A. Pandiscio, "Recording Skinfold Calipers for the Determination of Subcutaneous Edema," *J. Lab. and Clin. Med.*, 66, No. 1 (July 1965), 154–60.

219. Liddle, L., J. E. Seegmiller, and L. Laster, "The Enzymatic Spectrophotometric Method for Determination of Uric Acid," *J. Lab. and Clin. Med.*, 54 (December 1959), 903–13.

220. Lilienfeld, A. M., "Emotional and Other Characteristics of Cigarette Smokers and Nonsmokers as Related to Epidemiological Studies of Lung Cancer and Other Diseases," *J. Natl. Cancer Inst.*, 22, No. 2 (February 1959), 259–82.

221. Lloyd-Thomas, H. G., "The Exercise Electrocardiogram in Patients with Cardiac Pain," *British Heart Journal*, 23, No. 5 (September 1961), 561–77.

222. Lombard, W. P., and O. M. Cope, "The Duration of Systole in Man," *Amer. J. Physiol.*, 77, No. 2 (July 1926), 263–95.

223. Mack, P. B., "Bone Density Changes in the Astronauts During Flight," *Food and Nutrition News*, 40, No. 9 (June 1969), 1–4.

224. Marks, H. H., "Body Weight: Facts from the Life Insurance Records," in *Body Measurements and Human Nutrition*, J. Brozek, ed. Detroit: Wayne State University Press, 1956, 107–21.

225. ———, "Influence of Obesity on Morbidity and Mortality," *Bull. N.Y. Acad. Med.*, 36, No. 5 (May 1960), 296–312.

226. ———, "Relationship of Body Weight to Mortality and Morbidity," *Metabolism*, 6, No. 5 (September 1957), 417–24.

227. Mason, R. E., I. Likar, R. O. Biern, and R. S. Ross, "Multiple-Lead Exercise Electrocardiography. Experience in 107 Normal Subjects and 67 Patients with Angina Pectoris and Comparison with Coronary Cinearteriography in 84 Patients," *Circulation*, 36, No. 4 (October 1967), 517–25.

228. Mattingly, T. W., "The Post-Exercise Electrocardiogram. Its Value in the Diagnosis and Prognosis of Coronary Arterial Disease," *Amer. J. Cardiology*, 9, No. 3 (March 1962), 395–409.

229. Maxfield, M. E., "The Indirect Measurement of Energy Expenditure in Industrial Situations," *Amer. J. Clin. Nutrition*, 24, No. 9 (September 1971), 1126–38.

230. Mayer, J., "Exercise and Weight Control," Chap. 12, in *Exercise and Fitness*, S. C. Staley, ed. Chicago: The Athletic Institute, 1960.

231. ———, "Physical Activity and Anthropometric Measurements of Obese Adolescents," *Federation Proceedings*, 25, No. 1 (January–February 1966), 11–14.

232. ———, "The Role of Exercise and Activity in Weight Control," Chap. 17, in *Weight Control*. Ames, Ia.: Iowa State College Press, 1955.

233. McClean, C. E., P. C. Clason, and P. V. Stoughton, "The Peripheral Pulse as a Diagnostic Tool," *Angiology*, 15, No. 5 (May 1964), 221–31.

234. McConahay, D. R., C. M. Martin, M. D. Cheitlin, "Resting and Exercise Systolic Time Intervals: Correlations with Ventricular Performance in Patients with Coronary Artery Disease," *Circulation*, 45, No. 3 (March 1972), 592–601.

235. Metheny, E., L. Brouha, R. E. Johnson, and W. H. Forbes, "Some Physiologic Responses of Women and Men to Moderate and Strenuous Exercise: A Comparative Study," *Amer. J. Physiol.*, 137, No. 2 (September 1942), 318–26.

236. Metzger, C. C., F. W. Kroetz, and J. J. Leonard, "True Isovolumic Contraction Time and Its Correlation with Easily Measured External Indices of Ventricular Contractility (P)." *Circulation*, 36 (Supplement II) (October 1967), 187.

237. Miall, W. E., and P. D. Oldham, "Factors Influencing Arterial Blood Pressure in the General Population," *Clin. Sci.*, 17, No. 3 (1958), 409–40.

238. Mikkelsen, W. M., H. J. Dodge, and H. Valkenburg, "The Distribution of Serum Uric Acid Values in a Population Unselected as to Gout or Hyperuricemia: Tecumseh, Michigan, 1959–1960," *Amer. J. Med.*, 39, No. 2 (August 1965), 242–51.

239. Montoye, H. J., "Circulatory-Respiratory Fitness" in *An Introduction to Measurement in Physical Education, Vol. 4, Physical Fitness*, Henry J. Montoye, ed. Indianapolis: Phi Epsilon Kappa Fraternity, 1970, pp. 41–87.

240. ———, "Estimation of Habitual Physical Activity by Questionnaire and Interview," *Amer. J. Clinical Nutrition*, 24, No. 9 (September 1971), 1113–18.

241. ———, "Measurement of Body Fatness," Chap. 2, in *An Introduction to Measurement in Physical Education*, H. J. Montoye, ed. Indianapolis: Phi Epsilon Kappa Fraternity, 1970.

242. ———, "Physical Activity and Risk Factors Associated with Coronary Heart Disease," in *Exercise and Fitness*, B. D. Franks, ed. Chicago: Athletic Institute, 1969, pp. 43–52

243. ———, "The 'Harvard Step Test' and Work Capacity," *Revue canadienne de Biologie*, 11, No. 5 (March 1953), 491–99.

244. ———, "Vztah Obvyklé Tělesné Aktivity Ke Krevnímu Tlaku, Celkovému Cholesterolu v Séru a k Toleranci Glukózy," *Časopis Lékaru Českych*, 108, No. 41 (October 1969), 1216–20.

245. Montoye, H. J., D. A. Cunningham, H. G. Welch, and F. H. Epstein, "Laboratory Methods of Assessing Metabolic Capacity in a Large Epidemiological Study," *Amer. J. Epidemiol.*, 91, No. 1 (January 1970), 38–47.

246. Montoye, H. J., and F. H. Epstein, "Tecumseh Community Health Study: An Investigation of Health and Disease in an Entire Community," *J. Sports Med. and Phys. Fitness*, 5, No. 3 (September 1965), 127–31.

247. Montoye, H. J., F. H. Epstein, and M. O. Kjelsberg, "The Measurement of Body Fatness: A Study in a Total Community," *Amer. J. Clinical Nutrition*, 16, No. 5 (May 1965), 417–27.

248. Montoye, H. J., J. A. Faulkner, P. W. Willis III, W. D. Block, F. H. Epstein, H. J. Dodge, and W. M. Mikkelsen, "Serum Total Cholesterol Concentration in Business Executives: Intercorrelation with Physical Activity, Serum Uric Acid and Body Fatness." Proceedings, 16th World Congress of Sports Medicine. Koln-Berlin: Deutscher Arzteverlag, 1967.

249. Montoye, H. J., J. A. Faulkner, H. J. Dodge, W. M. Mikkelson, P. W. Willis

III, and W. D. Block, "Serum Uric Acid Concentration Among Business Executives: With Observations of Other Coronary Heart Disease Risk Factors," *Annals of Internal Medicine*, 66, No. 5 (May 1967), 838–50.

250. Montoye, H. J., M. E. Frantz, and A. J. Kozar, "The Value of Age, Height and Weight in Establishing Standards of Fitness for Children," *J. Sports Med. and Phys. Fitness*, 12, No. 3 (September 1972), 174–79.

251. Montoye, H. J., M. E. Frantz, A. J. Kozar, and B. C. Johnson, "Relation of Participation in Physical Education to Certain Clinical and Fitness Measurements," *Physical Educator*, 31, No. 1 (March 1974), 3–7.

252. Montoye, H. J., S. Guber, D. A. Cunningham, and S. Dinka, Jr., "Age and Acquisition of a 'Steady State' during Continuous, Graded Treadmill Exercise," *The Physiologist*, 13, No. 3 (August 1970), 263.

253. Montoye, H. J., G. E. Howard, and J. H. Wood, "Observations of Some Hemochemical and Anthropometric Measurements in Athletes," *J. Sports Med. and Phys. Fitness*, 7, No. 1 (March 1967), 35–44.

254. Montoye, H. J., H. L. Metzner, J. B. Keller, B. C. Johnson, and F. H. Epstein, "Habitual Physical Activity and Blood Pressure," *Medicine and Science in Sports*, 4, No. 4 (Winter 1972), 175–81.

255. Montoye, H. J., P. W. Willis III, D. A. Cunningham, and J. B. Keller, "Heart Rate Response to a Modified Harvard Step Test: Males and Females, Age 10–69," *Research Qtly.*, 40, No. 1 (March 1969), 153–62.

256. Montoye, H. J., P. W. Willis III, and D. A. Cunningham, "Heart Rate Response to Submaximal Exercise: Relation to Age and Sex," *J. Gerontol.*, 23, No. 2 (April 1968), 127–33.

257. Montoye, H. J., P. W. Willis III, G. E. Howard, and J. B. Keller, "Cardiac Preejection Period: Age and Sex Comparisons," *J. Gerontol.*, 26, No. 2 (April 1971), 208–16.

258. ———, "Systolic Preejection Period: Patients with Heart Disease Compared to Normal Subjects," *Archives of Environmental Health*, 28, No. 3 (September 1970), 425–31.

259. Montoye, H. J., P. W. Willis III, J. B. Keller, and H. L. Metzner, "Systolic Preejection Period: Relation to Habitual Physical Activity," *Medicine and Science in Sports*, 4, No. 2 (Summer 1972), 77–84.

260. Molnar, S., B. D. Franks, M. Jette, and T. K. Cureton, "Cardiac Time Components of Boys 7–14 Years of Age," *Medicine and Science in Sports*, 3, No. 1 (Spring 1971), 12–17.

261. Morris, J. N., "Epidemiology and Cardiovascular Disease of Middle Age: Part I," *Modern Concepts of Cardiovascular Disease*, 29 (1960), 625.

262. ———, *Uses of Epidemiology*. Baltimore: The Williams and Wilkins Co., 1964.

263. Morris, J. N., and M. D. Crawford, "Coronary Heart Disease and Physical Activity of Work," *Brit. Med. Journal*, 2 (December 20, 1958), 1485–96.

264. Mueller, E. F., S. V. Kasl, G. W. Brooks, and S. Cobb, "Psychosocial Correlates of Serum Urate Levels," *Psych. Bul.*, 73, No. 4 (April 1970), 238–57.

265. Murakami, N., S. Hori, and S. Masumura, "Exercise Proteinuria and Proteinuria Induced by Kallikrein," *Nature* (London), 218, No. 5140 (May 4, 1968), 481–83.

266. Nagle, F., B. Balke, G. Baptista, J. Alleyia, and E. Howley, "Compatability

of Progressive Treadmill, Bicycle, and Step Tests Based on Oxygen Uptake Responses," *Medicine and Science in Sports*, 3, No. 4 (Winter 1971), 149–54.

267. Nagle, F. J., B. Balke, and J. P. Naughton, "Gradational Step Tests for Assessing Work Capacity," *J. Appl. Physiol.*, 20, No. 4 (July 1965), 745–48.

268. Naimark, A., K. Wasserman, and M. B. McIlroy, "Continuous Measurement of Ventilatory Exchange Ratio During Exercise," *J. Appl. Physiol.*, 19, No. 4 (July 1964), 644–52.

269. Napier, J. A., "Field Methods and Response Rates in the Tecumseh Community Health Study," *Amer. J. Public Health*, 52, No. 2 (February 1962), 208–16.

270. Napier, J. A., B. C. Johnson, and F. H. Epstein, "The Tecumseh, Michigan Community Health Study," Chap. 2, in *The Community as an Epidemiologic Laboratory: A Casebook of Community Studies*, I. I. Kessler and M. L. Levin, eds. Baltimore: The Johns Hopkins Press, 1970, pp. 25–44.

271. Naughton, J., and W. Leach, "The Effect of a Simulated Warm-Up on Ventricular Performance," *Medicine and Science in Sports*, 3, No. 4 (Winter 1971), 169–71.

272. Nedbal, J., and V. Seliger, "Electrophoretic Analysis of Exercise Proteinuria," *J. Appl. Physiol.*, 13, No. 2 (September 1958), 244–58.

273. Neel, J. V., "The Clinical Detection of the Genetic Carriers of Inherited Disease," *Medicine*, 26, (May 1947), 115–53.

274. Nichols, J., A. T. Miller, Jr., and E. P. Hiatt, "Influence of Muscular Exercise on Uric Acid Excretion in Man," *J. Appl. Physiol.*, 3, No. 8 (February 1951), 501–7.

275. Nilsson, B. E., and N. E. Westlin, "Bone Density in Athletes," *Clinical Orthopaedics and Related Research*, 77 (1971), 179–82.

276. Norris, A. H., N. W. Shock, and M. J. Yiengst, "Age Changes in Heart Rate and Blood Pressure Response to Tilting and Standardized Exercise," *Circulation*, 8, No. 4 (October 1953), 521–26.

277. ————, "Age Differences in Ventilatory and Gas Exchange Responses to Graded Exercise in Males," *J. Gerontol.*, 10, No. 2 (April 1955), 145–55.

278. Novak, L. P., "Physical Activity and Body Composition of Adolescent Boys," *J. Amer. Med. Assn*, 197, No. 11 (September 12, 1966), 891–93.

279. *Obesity and Health.* U.S. Department of Health, Education and Welfare, Public Health Service Publication No. 1485. Washington, D.C.: U.S. Govt. Printing Office, 1966.

280. Ostman, I., and N. O. Sjöstrand, "Effect of Heavy Physical Training on the Catecholamine Content of the Heart and Adrenals of the Guinea Pig," *Experientia*, 27, No. 3 (March 1971), 270–71.

281. ————, "Effect of Prolonged Physical Training on the Catecholamine Levels of the Heart and the Adrenals of the Rat," *Acta Physiologica Scandinavica*, 82, No. 2 (June 1971), 202–8.

282. Otis, A. B., "Quantitative Relationships in Steady State Gas Exchange," in *Respiration, Vol. 1*, W. O. Fenn and H. Rahn, eds. Washington, D.C.: American Physiological Society, 1964, pp. 681–98.

283. Payne, M., and M. Kjelsberg, "Respiratory Symptoms, Lung Function, and Smoking Habits in an Adult Population," *Amer. J. Pub. Health*, 54, No. 2 (February 1964), 261–77.

284. Penpargkul, S., and J. Scheuer, "The Effect of Physical Training upon the Mechanical and Metabolic Performance of the Rat Heart," *J. Clinical Investigation*, 49, No. 10 (October 1970), 1859–68.

285. Perlman, L. V., D. Cunningham, H. Montoye, and B. Chiang, "Exercise Proteinuria," *Med. and Sci. in Sports*, 2, No. 1 (Spring 1970), 20–23.

286. Peterson, F. J., and D. L. Kelley, "The Effect of Cigarette Smoking upon the Acquisition of Physical Fitness During Training as Measured by Aerobic Capacity," *J. Amer. College Health Assn.*, 17, No. 3 (February 1969), 250–54.

287. Poortmans, J., and G. Lion, "Ultracentrifugation Analytique de la Proteinuric d'Effort," *Clinica Chemica Acts*, 8, No. 4 (July 1963), 632–34.

288. Price-Jones, C., D.B. Dill, and G.P. Wright, "The Concentration of Haemoglobin in Normal Human Blood," *J. Pathol. and Bacteriol.*, 34, No. 6 (November 1931), 779–87.

289. Puddu, V., A. Menotti, and H.W. Blackburn, "Observations on T Wave after Effort in Active and Sedentary Working Men," *Acta Cardiologia*, 20, No. 3 (1965), 210–17.

290. Quick, A. J., "The Effect of Exercise in the Excretion of Uric Acid," *J. Biolog. Chem.*, 110, No. 1 (June 1935), 107–12.

291. Raab, W., "Degenerative Heart Disease from Lack of Exercise," Chap. 2, in *Exercise and Fitness*. Chicago: Athletic Institute, 1960, pp. 10–19.

292. ———, ed., *Prevention of Ischemic Heart Disease*. Springfield, Ill.: Charles C Thomas, 1962.

293. ———, "The Adrenergic-Cholinergic Control of Cardiac Metabolism and Function," *Advanced Cardiology*, 1 (1956), 65–152.

294. ———, "Training, Physical Activity and the Cardiac Dynamic Cycle," *J. Sports Med. and Phys. Fitness*, 6, No. 1 (March 1966), 38–47.

295. Raab, W., E. de Paula, P. Silva, and Y. K. Starcheska, "Adrenergic and Cholinergic Influences in the Dynamic Cycle of the Normal Human Heart," *Cardiologia*, 33, No. 5 (1958), 350–64.

296. Raab, W., and W. Gigee, "Norepinephrine and Epinephrine Control of Normal and Diseased Human Hearts," *Circulation*, 11, No. 4 (April 1955), 593–603.

297. Raab, W., and H. J. Krzywank, "Cardiovascular Sympathetic Tone and Stress Response Related to Personality Patterns and Exercise Habits," *Amer. J. Cardiology*, 16, No. 1 (July 1965), 42–53.

298. Rahe, R. H., and R. J. Arthur, "Stressful Underwater Demolition Training," *J. Amer. Med. Assn.*, 202, No. 11 (December 11, 1967), 1052–54.

299. Rakestraw, N. W., "Chemical Factors in Fatigue. 1. The Effect of Muscular Exercise upon Certain Common Blood Constituents," *J. Biolog. Chem.*, 47, No. 3 (August 1921), 565–91.

300. Ramazzini, B., *De Morbis Artificum* (1713), W. C. Wright, trans. Chicago: The University of Chicago Press, 1940, p. 283.

301. Raven, P. B., T. J. Conners, and E. Evonuk, "Effects of Exercise on Plasma Lactic Dyhydrogenase Isozymes and Catecholamines," *J. Appl. Physiol.*, 29, No. 3 (September 1970), 374–77.

302. Raven, P. B., and E. Evonuk, "Plasma Catecholamines and Lactic Dehydrogenase Isozymes Following Exhaustive Exercise," *Physiologist*, 12, No. 3 (August 1969), 337.

303. Reedy, J. D., G. L. Saiger, and R. H. Hosler, "Evaluation of the Harvard Step Test with Respect to Factors of Height and Weight," *Internationale Zeitschrift Angewandte Physiologie*, 17, No. 2 (April 1958), 115–19.

304. Reiff, G. G., H. J. Montoye, R. D. Remington, J. A. Napier, H. L. Metzner, and F. H. Epstein, "Assessment of Physical Activity by Questionnaire and Interview," *J. Sports Med. and Phys. Fitness*, 7, No. 3 (September 1967), 135–42.

305. Reissman, L., "Class, Leisure and Social Participation," *American Sociological Review*, 19, No. 1 (February 1954), 76–84.

306. Remington, R. D., and A. Shork, "Determination of Number of Subjects Needed for Experimental Epidemiologic Studies of the Effect of Increased Physical Activity on Incidence of Coronary Heart Disease—Preliminary Considerations," in *Physical Activity and the Heart*, M. J. Karvonen and A. J. Barry, eds. Springfield, Ill.: Charles C Thomas, 1967, pp. 311–19.

307. Rennie, I. D. B., and H. Keen, "Evaluation of Clinical Methods of Detecting Proteinuria," *Lancet*, 2, No. 7514 (September 2, 1967), 489–92.

308. Rhyming, I., "A Modified Harvard Step Test for the Evaluation of Physical Fitness," *Arbeitsphysiologie*, 15, No. 4 (June 1954), 235–50.

309. Richardson, J. A., "Plasma Catecholamine in Angina Pectoris and Myocardial Infection," in *Prevention of Ischemic Heart Disease: Principles and Practices*, W. Raab, ed. Springfield, Ill.: Charles C Thomas, 1966, pp. 96–102.

310. Richardson, J. A., E. E. Woods, and E. E. Bagwell, "Circulatory Epinephrine and Norepinephrine in Coronary Occlusion," *Amer. J. Cardiology*, 5, No. 5 (May 1960), 613–18.

311. Robb, G. P., and H. H. Marks, "Post-Exercise Electrocardiogram in Arteriosclerotic Heart Disease," *J. Amer. Med. Assn.*, 200, No. 11 (June 2, 1967), 918–26.

312. Robbins, S. L., *Pathology*, 3rd ed. Philadelphia: W. B. Saunders Co., 1967, p. 228.

313. Robinson, J. A., H. I. C. Wong, H. T. Shelby, and D. J. Liv, "Preliminary Studies of the Effect of Exercise on Plasma Catecholamines of Cockrels. *Federation Proceedings*, 26, No. 2 (April 1967), 494.

314. Robinson, S., "Experimental Studies of Physical Fitness in Relation to Age," *Arbeitsphysiologie*, 10, No. 3 (October 1938), 251–323.

315. ———, "The Regulation of Sweating in Exercise," Chap. 9, in *Advances in Biology of Skin*, Vol. III. London: Pergamon Press, 1962.

316. Robinson, S., D. L. Mountjoy, and R. W. Bullard, "Influence of Fatigue on the Efficiency of Men During Exhausting Runs," *J. Appl. Physiol.*, 12, No. 2 (March 1958), 197–201.

317. Rose, G., "Physical Activity and Coronary Heart Disease in Symposium on the Meaning of Physical Fitness," *Proceedings of the Royal Society of Medicine*, 62 (November 1969), 1183–88.

318. Rosenman, R. H., "The Role of a Specific Overt Behavior Pattern in the Genesis of Coronary Heart Disease," in *Prevention of Ischemic Heart Disease: Principles and Practices*, W. Raab, ed. Springfield, Ill.: Charles C Thomas, 1966, pp. 201–207.

319. Rumball, C. A., and E. D. Acheson, "Electrocardiograms of Healthy Men After Strenuous Exercise," *British Heart Journal*, 22 (June 1960), 415–25.

320. Runes, D. D., and T. Kierman, eds. *Hippocrates. The Theory and Practice of Medicine.* New York: Philosophical Library, 1964, p. 17.

321. Saiki, H., R. Margaria, and F. Cuttica, "Lactic Acid Production in Submaximal Work," *Internationale Zeitschrift für Angewandt Physiologie Einschliesslich Arbeitsphysiologie,* 24, No. 1 (May 22, 1967), 57–61.

322. Saltzman, S. H., H. K. Hellerstein, J. H. Bruell, and D. Starr, "Adaptations to Muscular Exercise: The Effects on Epinephrine Induced Myocardial Necrosis in C34 Mice," *Circulation,* Supplement VI (October 1968), 170.

323. Saltzman, S. H., E. Z. Hirsch, H. K. Hellerstein, and J. H. Bruell, "Adaptations to Muscular Exercise: Myocardial Epinephrine—3H Uptake," *J. Appl. Physiol.,* 29, No. 1 (July 1970), 92–95.

324. Scheur, J., and S. W. Stezoski, "The Effect of Physical Conditioning on the Cardiac Response to Hypoxia," *J. Lab. and Clin. Med.,* 78, No. 5 (November 1971), 806–7.

325. Schwalb, H., "Unterschungen über die Okonomie und Leistungsfahigkeit des Kreislaufs im mittleren Lebensalter," *Archiv Für Kreislaufforschung 56,* No. 3–4 (August 1968), 151–235.

326. Scott, M. G., and E. French, *Evaluation in Physical Education.* St. Louis: C. V. Mosby Co., 1950.

327. Seltzer, C., "Anthropometric Characteristics and Physical Fitness," *Research Qtly,* 17, No. 1 (March 1946), 10–20.

328. Selye, H., "The Role of Stress in the Production and Prevention of Experimental Cardiopathies," in *Prevention of Ischemic Heart Disease: Principles and Practices,* W. Raab, ed. Springfield, Ill.: Charles C Thomas, 1966, pp. 163–68.

329. Shephard, R. J., "Comments on 'Cardiac Frequency in Relation to Aerobic Capacity for Work,'" *Ergonomics,* 13, No. 4 (1970), 509–13.

330. Shkhvatsagaya, I. K., "Experimental Production of Myocardial Lesions by Disturbing the Central Nervous System," in *Prevention of Ischemic Heart Disease: Principles and Practices,* W. Raab, ed. Springfield, Ill.: Charles C Thomas, 1966, pp. 39–48.

331. Simonson, E., *Differentiation Between Normal and Abnormal Electrocardiography.* St. Louis: C. V. Mosby Co., 1961, p. 191.

332. ———, "Physical Fitness and Work Capacity of Older Men," *Geriatrics,* 2, No. 2 (March–April 1947), 110–19.

333. ———, *Physiology of Work Capacity and Fatigue.* Springfield, Ill.: Charles C Thomas, 1971.

334. Sloan, A. W., "Physical Fitness of College Students in South Africa, United States of America, and England," *Research Qtly,* 34, No. 2 (May 1963), 244–48.

335. Sloan, N., and M. Liba, "The Effects of Participation in Physical Education on Achievement in Selected Characteristics," *Research Qtly,* 37, No. 3 (October 1966), 410–23.

336. Snellen, J. W., "Body Temperature During Exercise," *Medicine and Science in Sports,* 1, No. 1 (March 1969), 39–42.

337. Somogyi, M., "Determination of Blood Sugar," *J. Biolog. Chem.,* 160, No. 1 (September 1945), 69.

338. Sosna, A., "The Influence of Fencing on the Limb Musculature," in *Physical*

Fitness and Its Laboratory Assessment, J. Kral and V. Novotny, eds. Prague: Universita Karlova, 1970, pp. 80–83.

339. Spain, D. M., and D. J. Nathan, "Smoking Habits and Coronary Atherosclerotic Heart Disease," *J. Amer. Med. Assn.*, 177, No. 10 (September 1961), 683–88.

340. Stamler, J., D. M. Berkson, Q. D. Young, H. A. Lindberg, Y. Hall, W. Miller, and R. Stamler, "Approaches to the Prevention of Coronary Heart Disease," *J. Amer. Diabetic Assn.*, 40, No. 5 (May 1962), 407–16.

341. Stamler, J., Q. D. Young, Y. Hall, and S. L. Andelman, "Diet and Serum Lipids in Atherosclerotic Coronary Heart Disease," *Medical Clinics of North America* (January 1963), 3–31.

342. Starcich, R., "Plasma Catecholamines and Urinary Vanillyl Mandelic Acid in Clinical Ischemic Heart Disease," in *Prevention of Ischemic Heart Disease: Principles and Practices*, W. Raab, ed. Springfield, Ill.: Charles C Thomas, 1966, pp. 103–11.

343. Starr, I., "An Essay on the Strength of the Heart and on the Effect of Aging Upon It," *Amer. J. Cardiology*, 14, No. 6 (December 1964), 771–83.

344. Stetten, D., Jr., "Gout," *Perspectives in Biology and Medicine*, 2, No. 2 (Winter 1959), 185–96.

345. Stetten, D., Jr., and J. Z. Hearon, "Intellectual Level Measured by Army Classification Battery and Serum Uric Acid Concentration," *Science*, 129, No. 3365 (June 1959), 1737.

346. Strandell, T., "Electrocardiographic Findings at Rest, During and After Exercise in Healthy Old Men Compared with Young Men," *Acta Medica Scandinavica*, 174, No. 4 (October 1963), 479–99.

347. Sutton, G. C., S. M. Little, and J. McClung, "Measurements of Mechanical and Electrical Events of the Cardiac Cycle: Effect of Tachycardia, Pre-Anesthetic Medication and Di-ethyl Ether Anesthetics," *Amer. J. Med. Sc.*, 232, No. 6 (December 1956), 648–53.

348. Sutton-Smith, B., J. M. Roberts and R. M. Kozelka, "Game Involvement in Adults," *J. Soc. Psych.*, 60 (June 1963), 15–30.

349. Talley, R. C., J. F. Meyer, and J. L. McKay, "Evaluation of the Pre-Ejection Period as an Estimate of Myocardial Contractility in Dogs," *Amer. J. Cardiology*, 27, No. 4 (April 1971), 384–91.

350. Taylor, A. W., J. H. Schueman, A. R. Esfandiary, and J. C. Russell, "Effect of Exercise in Urinary Catecholamine Excretion in Active and Sedentary Subjects," *Révue canadienne de Biologie*, 30, No. 2 (June 1971), 97–105.

351. Taylor, H. L., "Occupational Factors in the Study of Coronary Heart Disease and Physical Activity," *Canad. Med. Assn. Journal*, 96, No. 12 (March 25, 1967), 825–31.

352. Taylor, H. L., H. Blackburn, C. L. V. Puchner, R. W. Parlin, and A. Keys, "Coronary Heart Disease in Selected Occupations of American Railroads in Relation to Physical Activity," *Circulation*, Supplement III, 40 (November 13–16, 1969), 202.

353. Taylor, H. L., E. Buskirk, B. Balke, H. Blackburn, and R. Remington, "Relationship of Adherence in a Supervised Physical Activity Program to Change in CHD Risk Factors and Work Capacity," *Circulation*, 46, No. 4 (October 1972), II–12.

354. Taylor, H. L., R. W. Parlin, H. Blackburn, and A. Keys, "Problems in the

Analysis of the Relationship of Coronary Heart Disease to Physical Activity or Its Lack, with Special Reference to Sample Size and Occupational Withdrawal," in *Physical Activity in Health and Disease*, K. Evang and K. L. Anderson, eds. Baltimore: The Williams and Wilkins Co., 1966, pp. 242–61.

355. Technicon Laboratory. *Autoanalyzer Method for Serum Uric Acid Determination.* Chauncey, N.Y., 1963.

356. "Tecumseh Community Health Study," *Research News*, (Office of Research Administration, The University of Michigan), 12, No. 12 (June 1, 1962), 1–4.

357. "Tecumseh Community Health Study," *Reasearch News*, Office of Research Administration, The University of Michigan, 19, No. 2 (August 1968), 1–6.

358. Tepperman, J., "Adipose Tissue: Yang and Yin," in *Fat as a Tissue*, K. Rodahl and B. Issekutz, eds. New York: McGraw-Hill, 1964, pp. 394–409.

359. Tharp, G. D., "Cardiac Function Tests as Indexes of Fitness," *Research Qtly.*, 40, No. 4 (December 1969), 818–22.

360. Thomas, C. B., "Characteristics of Smokers Compared with Nonsmokers in a Population of Healthy Young Adults, Including Observations on Family History, Blood Pressure, Heart Rate, Body Weight, Cholesterol and Certain Psychological Traits," *Ann. Internal Med.*, 53, No. 4 (October 1960), 697–718.

361. ———, "The Precursors of Hypertension," *Medical Clinics of North America*, 45, No. 2 (March 1961), 259–69.

362. Thomasson, G. O., "Serum Uric Acid as a Predictor of Athletic Achievement." Presented at the 16th Annual Meeting of the American College of Sports Medicine, Atlanta, Georgia, 1969.

363. Wasserman, K., A. L. VanKessel, and G. G. Burton, "Interaction of Physiological Mechanisms During Exercise," *J. Appl. Physiol.*, 22, No. 1 (January 1967), 71–85.

364. Webb, P., and U. C. Luft, "The Cumulative Oxygen of Continuous Work," *Federation Proceedings*, 30, No. 2 (March–April 1971), 371.

365. Welham, W. C., and A. R. Behnke, "Specific Gravity of Healthy Men. Body Weight ÷ Volume and Other Physical Characteristics of Exceptional Athletes and of Naval Personnel," *J. Amer. Med. Assn.*, 118, No. 7 (February 14, 1942), 495–501.

366. Weissler, A. M., "The Heart in Heart Failure," *Ann. Internal Med.*, 69, No. 5 (November 1968), 928–40.

367. Weissler, A. M., W. S. Harris, and C. D. Shoenfield, "Systolic Time Intervals in Heart Failure in Man," *Circulation*, 37, No. 2 (February 1968), 149–59.

368. Weissler, A. M., L. C. Harris, and G. D. White, "Left Ventricular Ejection Time in Man," *J. Appl. Physiol.*, 18, No. 5 (September 1963), 919–23.

369. Weissler, A. M., R. G. Peller, and W. H. Roehll, "Relationships between Left Ventricular Ejection Time, Stroke Volume, and Heart Rate in Normal Individuals and Patients with Cardiovascular Disease," *Amer. Heart Journal*, 62, No. 3 (September 1961), 367–68.

370. Wessel, J., H. J. Montoye, and H. Mitchel, "Physical Activity Assessment by Recall Record," *Amer. J. Pub. Health*, 55, No. 9 (September 1965), 1430–36.

371. Whipp, B. J., and K. Wasserman, "Oxygen Uptake Kinetics for Various Intensities of Constant-Load Work," *J. Appl. Physiol.*, 33, No. 3 (September 1972), 351–56.

372. White, R. C., "Social Class Differences in the Use of Leisure," *Amer. J. Sociol.*, 61, No. 2 (September 1955), 145–50.

373. Whitsett, T., and J. Naughton, "The Effect of Exercise on Systolic Time Intervals in Sedentary and Active Individuals and Rehabilitated Patients with Heart Disease," *Amer. J. Cardiology*, 27, No. 4 (April 1971), 352–58.

374. Whitsett, T., J. Naughton, and M. T. Lategola, "The Response of Ventricular Ejection Time to Exercise in Patients with Atherosclerotic Heart Disease," *Abstract.* 16th Annual Meeting, American College of Sports Medicine, 1969.

375. Wiley, J. F., "Effects of 10 Weeks of Endurance Training on Left Ventricular Intervals," *J. Sports Med. and Phys. Fitness*, 11, No. 2 (June 1971), 104–11.

376. Winters, W. G., D. M. Leaman, and R. A. Anderson, "The Effect of Exercise on the Systolic Time Intervals in Men," *Circulation*, 46, No. 4 (October 1972), II–62.

377. Wolferth, C. C., and A. Margolies, "Asynchronism in Contraction of the Ventricles in the So-Called Common Type of Bundle–Branch Block: Its Bearing on the Determination of the Site of the Significant Lesion and on the Mechanism of Split First and Second Heart Sounds," *Amer. Heart Journal*, 10, No. 4 (April 1935), 425–58.

378. Wurtman, R. J., I. J. Kopin, and J. Axelrod, "Thyroid Function and the Cardiac Disposition of Catecholamines," *Endocrinology*, 73, No. 1 (July 1963), 63–74.

379. *Youth Fitness Test Manual.* Washington, D.C.: American Association for Health, Physical Education, and Recreation, 1962.

380. Zachau-Christiansen, B., "The Rise in the Serum Uric Acid during Muscular Exercise," *Scandanavian J. Clin. Lab. Investigation*, 11, No. 1 (January 1959), 57–60.

381. Zborowski, M., and L. Eyde, "Aging and Social Participation," *J. Gerontol.*, 17, No. 4 (October 1962), 424–30.

382. Zoethout, D., and W. W. Tuttle, *Textbook of Physiology.* St. Louis: C. V. Mosby Co., 1952, p. 703.

Index